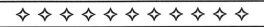

Madness, Heresy, and the Rumor of Angels

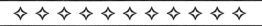

Madness, Heresy, and the Rumor of Angels

The Revolt against the Mental Health System

Seth Farber

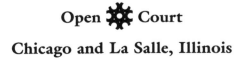

Open **✼** Court

Chicago and La Salle, Illinois

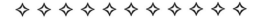

Front cover illustration: *The Angel of the Flowing Light* by
Cecil Collins, 1968. Oil on board. Reproduced by permission
of The Tate Gallery, London.

OPEN COURT and the above logo are registered in the U.S.
Patent and Trademark Office.

©1993 by Open Court Publishing Company

First printing 1993

Printed and bound in the United States of America.

Library of Congress Cataloging-in-Publication Data
Farber, Seth, 1951–
    Madness, heresy, and the rumor of angels : the revolt against
the mental health system / Seth Farber.
        p.   cm.
    Includes bibliographical references and index.
    ISBN 0-8126-9199-7. — ISBN 0-8126-9200-4 (paper)
    1. Antipsychiatry. 2. Psychotherapy patients—Abuse of.
3. Ex-mental patients—Case studies.   I. Title.
RC437.5.F35   1993
616.89—dc20   93-1276
                                                          CIP

This book is dedicated to those psychiatric survivors who have refused to accept their 'psychiatric diagnoses'—and have thereby affirmed our common humanity.

A spiritualised society would treat in its sociology the individual, from the saint to the criminal, not as units of a social problem to be passed through some skilfully devised machinery and either flattened into the social mould or crushed out of it, but as souls suffering and entangled in a net and to be rescued, souls growing and to be encouraged to grow, souls grown and from whom help and power can be drawn by the lesser spirits who are not yet adult. The aim of its economics would be not to create a huge engine of production, whether of the competitive or the co-operative kind, but to give to men—not only to some but to all men each in his highest possible measure—the joy of work according to their own nature and free leisure to grow inwardly, as well as a simply rich and beautiful life for all. In its politics it would not regard the nations within the scope of their own internal life as enormous State machines regulated and armoured with man living for the sake of the machine and worshipping it as his God and his larger self, content at the first call to kill others upon its altar and to bleed there himself so that the machine may remain intact and powerful and be made ever larger, more complex, more cumbrous, more mechanically efficient and entire. Neither would it be content to maintain these nations or States in their mutual relations as noxious engines meant to discharge poisonous gas upon each other in peace and to rush in times of clash upon each other's armed hosts and unarmed millions, full of belching shot and men missioned to murder like hostile tanks in a modern battlefield. It would regard the peoples as group-souls, the Divinity concealed and to be self-discovered in its human collectivities, group-souls meant like the individual to grow according to their own nature and by that growth to help each other, to help the whole race in the one common work of humanity. And that work would be to find the divine Self in the individual and the collectivity and to realise spiritually, mentally, vitally, materially its greatest, largest, richest and deepest possibilities in the inner life of all and their outer action and nature.

—SRI AUROBINDO

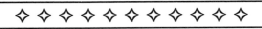

Contents

✧ ✧ ✧ ✧ ✧ ✧ ✧

Part I: Lunatics, Lovers, and Poets

✧ ✧ ✧ ✧ ✧ ✧ ✧

Part II: Heretics, Apostates, and Infidels

✧ ✧ ✧ ✧ ✧ ✧ ✧ ✧ ✧ ✧ ✧

Foreword

This book presents the tragic tale of seven persons who sought psychiatric help, and found psychiatric harm. Why did this happen? Whose fault was it? Seth Farber blames psychiatry. I agree. However, although I consider psychiatry's guilt for misinforming people and mangling their lives self-evident, I also hold the victims partly responsible for their fate. Why? Because I believe it is every person's responsibility to inform himself, to the best of his ability, about the world he lives in. "A popular government without popular information, or the means of acquiring it," warned James Madison, "is but a prologue to a farce, or a tragedy, or perhaps both. Knowledge will forever govern ignorance; and people who mean to be their own governors, must arm themselves with the power which knowledge gives."

Madison's remarks about *political* self-government apply with even greater force to *personal* self-government, especially in a modern society in which the manipulation of information is of paramount importance. The less a person knows about the workings of the social institutions of his society, the more he must trust those who wield power in it; and the more he trusts those who wield such power, the more vulnerable he makes himself to becoming their victim. No one who has read or seen Ken Kesey's *One Flew Over the Cuckoo's Nest*—or similar stories about psychiatry, going back to Chekhov's classic *Ward No. 6*—can claim to be ignorant of the dangers mad-doctors pose to every man, woman, and child in America. How can this be? Psychiatrists are physicians, and physicians are supposed to help people. That is true. But it does not follow that the result is necessarily helpful for the so-called patient—as he, the patient, would define what constitutes help.

I began by making a doubly unfashionable assertion, which I would now like to amplify. I suggested that both the psychiatric victimizer *and* his victim must share the blame—though not necessarily in equal proportion—for the injury the former inevitably inflicts on the latter. However, the men and women whose story Farber tells—and a few others who, sadly, represent a small minority—are also responsible for saving themselves in the end. Unlike the typical victim of psychiatric despotism who comes to love his oppressor and to believe in the oppressor's goodness, these seven had the courage and good sense to learn from their experience, escape from psychiatric slavery, and shed their illusions about the benevolence of jailers and poisoners who masquerade as doctors.

The institution of psychiatry—epitomized by the practice of incarcerating persons innocent of crimes in buildings deceptively called 'hospitals'—has always been dangerous to the welfare of its inmates. It had never been the purpose of psychiatry to help the inmates rendered powerless by psychiatric imprisonment. Psychiatry's aim has always been, and still is, to help a relatively more powerful person—primarily the denominated patient's parent, spouse, or other relative—by disqualifying his less powerful kin whose behavior troubles him as 'troubled', which is to say mad, and by incarcerating the victim defined as a 'patient' in a madhouse. While this has always been true, it seems to me that Americans today are more misinformed and more gullible about the true nature of psychiatry than people anywhere have ever been. Accordingly, it is imperative that men, women, and children learn to protect themselves from the dangers of psychiatry. As adolescents must learn not to swim on beaches where the undertow is powerful, lest they be unable to make it back to shore, and not to climb mountains during a thunderstorm, lest they be struck by lightning, they must also learn, when their lives are stormy, to avoid psychiatrists and stay away from mental hospitals, as the only buildings in America they can enter, but not leave, voluntarily.

For as far back as I can remember, it has seemed to me self-evident that people who have knowledge and skill do not need power to coerce others; that people who have power are *ipso facto* dangerous to others; that, as Lord Acton warned, "Power tends to corrupt, and absolute power corrupts absolutely"; that, because of the obvious connections between power and evil, only the corrupt seek power, and the most corrupt seek the most absolute power; in short, that when a person goes for help he must always be mindful of the old Roman adage, *caveat emptor* (buyer beware). Because psychiatrists have a great deal of power, and because they are utterly corrupted by the pretense of helping so-called patients while in fact acting as agents of social control on behalf of the patients' familial and social antagonists, it is imperative that potential consumers of psychiatric services be familiar not with what mental health professionals *say,* but with what they *do.*

One of the most remarkable facts of life is that, of all the creatures on Earth, none is more supportive of members of its own species than man—*and* more destructive towards them. The ostensible mandate of all of our major social institutions—family, church, medicine, the state—is to help people. Yet, each of these institutions, and the individuals who implement their workings, can also pose the gravest threat to our life, liberty, and health.

Farber's reconstruction of the encounters of seven persons with their psychiatric malefactors demonstrates, through the voices of the victims, the tragic misunderstandings between persons seeking psychiatric help and psychiatrists ostensibly dispensing it. I say "tragic misunderstandings", because six out of seven of the psychiatric victims who speak to us through these pages ventured *voluntarily* into the labyrinth where mad-doctors manufacture madness. What did they expect from the psychiatrists? Did they understand the professional job-description of these fake doctors? Did they understand that the doors of mental hospitals can, at any moment, be locked by the psychiatrists, trapping the patients inside? And that, thenceforth, the prisoner's wish to leave the prison called 'hospital' will medically and legally justify keeping him confined? If they did not know these things, why didn't they? Didn't they realize that psychiatrists have the power to commit and confine people and hence, unless they renounce that power—which no hospital psychiatrist does, or indeed could do—the psychiatrists are, *ipso facto,* not their patients' agents? Didn't these victims of psychiatry ever hear the maxim, 'He who pays the piper calls the tune'?

Let us look behind the curtain that conceals the inner workings of psychiatric victimization. It is not difficult to do that. However, it requires that we accept the reality of man's humanity *and* inhumanity to man, and that we ask ourselves some basic questions, such as: What do we mean when we say we *help* a person? What *counts* as help? Who *defines* what counts as help?

If the helpless person is an infant, the answer is relatively simple: Help is food, shelter, the love of parents or parent-substitutes. If the helpless person is an adult, the answers can be agonizingly uncertain and hopelessly controversial. Consider some illustrative scenarios.

A man complains of abdominal pain. How do we help him? Should we simply do what he asks us to do? Perhaps. But suppose all he says is: 'Help me!' Should we give him a drug to relieve his pain? Should we remove his appendix—because that is what is causing his pain? Should we kill him—because he is suffering from a rapidly spreading cancer which is causing his pain? Should we advise him to commit suicide? Should we pray for him.

A man is hungry. How do we help him? As Confucius taught us, we can help him by giving him a fish or by teaching him how to fish. Do we help him if we feed him and thus make him dependent on us? Do we help him if we refuse to feed him and thus compel him to choose between independence and starvation? It will not do to say that it all depends on circumstances, on the helpless person's ability or inability to help himself. While true, saying it merely exempts us from making a decision *now.*

A person is confused, troubled, agitated, feels guilty, cannot sleep, suspects others of evil deeds. How do we help an Othello, consumed with jealousy? A Hamlet, half out of his mind with the suspicion that his mother and uncle have murdered his father? A Lady Macbeth, maddened by the memory of her murderous deeds?

These are not scientific questions, not medical questions, not questions about what the best psychiatric treatment is for one or another so-called mental illness. They are riddles about life. People have struggled with these questions since ancient times. The best moral rule medical ethicists of antiquity could come up with was: *Primum non nocere* (First, do no harm). This sounds better than it is. For the questions still remain: What is harm? What is help? To complicate matters, since human beings manipulate symbols with infinite inventivenss, the propensity to harm people in the name of helping them is one of mankind's favorite occupations.

I do not doubt that the desire to help is often genuine. The problem is that, if the Other's affliction lies in his soul rather than his body, then our urge to help him cannot be satisfied without our feeling empathy for him, indeed, without our establishing a bond of intimacy with him. This is why helping people *impersonally*—for example, by shipping food or medicine to victims of wars or natural disasters—can be organized; but helping persons *personally*—*qua* individuals—cannot be organized. Of course, this has not prevented people from trying to organize such help. Inevitably, the very attempt turns into a disaster, into an opportunity for existential cannibalism. I use this term to denote encounters officially defined as therapeutic that, in fact, consist of the malefactor de-meaning his maleficiary —by destroying the meaning that he, the nominal beneficiary, has given his own existence. There are many ways of practicing existential cannibalism. In our society, the most popular form of it is to give one's 'beneficiary' a psychiatric diagnosis and impose on him a psychiatric treatment, neither of which he wants. This enables the 'benefactor' to claim he is helping and strengthening his 'beneficiary', while, in fact, he is harming him and is rendering him more powerless.

Farber's book is a useful counterpoise to the mental health industry's massive campaign of disinformation, essential for maintaining the practice of psychiatric cannibalism. For every patient psychiatrists claim to have helped, Farber can show us one who claims he has been harmed. Against every glamor story about the therapeutic powers of neuroleptic drugs, electric shocks, and incarceration in insane asylums told by psychiatrists, Farber can pit a horror story about the noxious powers of psychiatrists exercised by means of their deceptive vocabulary and pseudomedical interventions. In short, Farber's book depicts what he and I—and perhaps a silent minority of Americans —regard as the psychiatric professions's most distinguishing feature, namely, the deliberate, systematic dehumanization of man, in the name of mental health.

Federal law now requires that drugs—for example, alcohol and cigarettes—carry a warning label, cautioning the buyer about the risks he assumes if he uses the product. It is not a new idea. After all, Dante had depicted the entrance to Hell as emblazoned with the warning: "All hope abandon, ye who enter here!" Not until the same warning is prominently displayed over the office door of every mental health professional who has not forsworn therapeutic coercion, and over the entrance to every mental hospital, will persons who contemplate seeking psychiatric help be in a position to give informed consent to their social stigmatization and spiritual self-destruction.

Thomas Szasz

Preface

Readers may wonder how I chose the individuals whose stories I tell in this book. Several I met through the anti-psychiatry movement. Others were among a large number of persons who contacted me after hearing me on T.V. or the radio. I did not preselect subjects to confirm my thesis that madness is an intrinsically spiritual experience. I believe that my subjects are a representative sample of former 'mental patients'. They are distinguished from most of their peers not by their spirituality, but by two significant traits. They are more skeptical of authority, more independently-minded than the average psychiatric survivor, which explains why they rebelled against the mental health system and extricated themselves from it. Second they probably have more education or self-education, and consequently more developed verbal skills, than the average psychiatric survivor—or the average person. I deliberately chose unusually articulate persons to interview.

Many of my critics no doubt will attempt to discredit my arguments by insisting that these individuals are exceptional and hence that their stories do not invalidate psychiatry's claim that 'schizophrenia' and other 'severe mental disorders' are chronic and debilitating. But as their accounts make clear, all of them manifested the behaviors typically construed by psychiatrists as symptoms of severe mental illnesses. These individuals are exceptional primarily in the sense that they are forerunners and that they can and will serve as role models for other psychiatric survivors who will follow their example and refuse to allow mental health professionals to destroy their dignity and induct them into careers as professional mental patients.

I make no attempt to disguise or apologize for my unfashionable view that there is a transcendental, spiritual reality, and that many experiences dismissed as 'delusional' are glimpses of that reality. But it is not necessary to share my religious outlook in order to share my abhorrence of the mental health system. You need not accept the veridicality or religious validity of my subjects' experiences in order to defend their right not to be involuntarily incarcerated and coercively 'treated'. Emmanuel

Swedenborg, the Swedish mystic, claimed to have daily conversations with angels and other spirits. A skeptic might doubt this claim and still respect this man who was a renowned theologian and a prolific writer, and who was never menaced with the threat of psychiatric incarceration. Some skeptics may go farther, and view with disdain all mystical experiences, regarding those persons who report such experiences as highly fanciful and somewhat foolish. Yet still, we can hopefully at least agree to reject the supposition that everyone who thinks and feels differently from you or me ought *ipso facto* to be classified as medically sick and as a candidate to be locked up and abused. An atheist paraphrasing Voltaire might say to one of my subjects: 'I don't agree with a word you say, but I will defend to the death your right to say it without being disqualified as mentally ill.'

Why were six of my seven subjects women? I do not know. Perhaps it is because woman survivors of psychiatric incarceration are more ready than male survivors to disenthrall themselves from a system that represents a monstrous abuse of male power. One might speculate that this is one manifestation of a phenomenon that is cosmic in its dimensions. Nature—the Earth itself—is rising from her torpor to demand recognition of her claim to sanctity, to insist on the acceptance of her right to be reverenced. (Other manifestations of this phenomenon would be ecological movements and the animal rights movement.)

Finally, I want to thank those over the years who helped me complete my projects. I want to thank my parents for their support and confidence. I want to thank Stewart Miller for encouraging me to write this book and unwittingly inspiring the title. I want to thank Leonard Frank, Don Weitz, Thomas Szasz, Monty Weinstein, Jack Felder, Carol Lorenzo, Judith Greenberg, Caren Santiz, Peter Breggin, and Kate Millett, and all the people interviewed herein for their time and patience. I want to thank David Ramsay Steele for his wise suggestions, Laura Woodruff for her perspicacity and patience, Joe Pavia for organizing the troops, Charmaine Tyson for her intelligence and kindness, and Lisa DeVito for the rainbow she revealed and the flame she lit.

Seth Farber

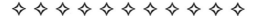

Introduction

"I saw the best minds of my generation destroyed by madness," wrote Allen Ginsberg in *Howl*. I believe this statement is inaccurate: I contend that he saw the best minds of his generation destroyed by the 'mental health' system. Contrary to popular opinion (encouraged by a formidable public-relations campaign) the mental health system has not changed significantly since Ginsberg wrote *Howl* in the 1950s. But there has been one rather significant change since Ginsberg saw his friends destroyed: at least *some* of the best minds of *my* generation have survived this system. They triumphed. This book tells how and why.

As to madness, most of the psychiatric survivors I interviewed (and others with militant viewpoints I've spoken to) agree with the late psychiatrist R.D. Laing: 'madness', however painful it may be, can provide the opportunity to re-create one's self and expand one's possibilities. In their time of madness the subjects interviewed here became aware of the 'spiritual' dimension of human existence; they experienced their oneness with all beings.

I have interviewed and told here the story of seven individuals. If we could look at their 'case records' we would be able to verify that they were classified by the numerous professionals who 'treated' them as 'chronically mentally ill'. Each person was typically given various diagnoses by different professionals: 'schizophrenic', 'manic-depressive' ('bipolar disorder'), 'borderline personality disorder', and so forth. From the point of view of the mental health expert, they were clearly severely mentally ill. The 'expert' would say they are still ill or that their illness is 'in remission'. They exhibited the 'symptoms' that typically warrant the diagnosis of schizophrenia or manic-depression. Yet they do not conform to the mental health experts' expectations: they are not taking psychiatric drugs, collecting disability funds from the government, or manifesting an inability to work and form intimate relationships. To the contrary, those individuals are leaders: keenly aware of the inequities in society, highly socially responsible and strongly determined to change the world, to save the Earth, and to redress injustice.

1

A sequence of events and experiences can be *storied* in a variety of different fashions. The *meaning* of these events is determined by the particular narrative ploys and metaphors that we utilize in order to shape and organize these events, by the way in which the raw material of life is configured. In order to demonstrate this to the reader I decided to construct two competing narrative lines for each subject I interviewed.

The dominant narrative line was the product of the fusion of my psyche with that of the subject. Each person interviewed felt that the narrative line which emerged did justice to the complexity of their experience and to the mystery of their soul's quest for meaning and fulfillment. The narrative line I counterpoised to this is one standardly constructed by mental health experts. On the one hand is the experts' case study of a damaged individual afflicted with the symptoms of mental illness. On the other hand is the story that seemed evident to me, the story of quest, of descent into madness, of spiritual vision, of existential crisis, of triumph, of self-discovery and spiritual transformation.

This format enables the reader to see how 'mental illness' stories are constructed and how they come to acquire their plausibility. It allows the reader to compare and judge for himself or herself: Is this officially sanctioned story the Truth? Or is it a banal and demeaning way of *storying* the events and experiences in a person's life? Many readers will be led to ponder the next logical question: Why do we continue to place our trust in a community of experts who have become skilled in construing and interpreting events in such a way that they fail to do justice to the dignity of the individual and to the value of the human quest for meaning and happiness?

This format forces readers to experience *themselves* the desecration of the human spirit involved in the 'mental health' enterprise. At times this will be an aggravating or painful process for the reader. Those experiences that are most *intimate* to the individual cannot be communicated to mental health professionals who work in mental hospitals without risking the violation of the self. On the one hand the most precious and inspiring experiences the individual has and on the other hand those experiences that reveal most starkly the individual's human vulnerability are typically not understood or appreciated by mental health experts. On the contrary it is these experiences that are most likely to be seized upon and interpreted as proof of the individual's 'psychopathology'.

My purpose is not primarily to entertain. It is to jar and disturb the reader as well as to awaken his or her reverence for the indomitability of the human spirit. Hopefully, the perspective presented here will inspire the reader and give to him or her an enhanced sense of human possibility.

PART ONE

Lunatics, Lovers, and Poets

Lovers and madmen have such
*   seething brains,*
Such shaping fantasies, that
*   apprehend*
More than cool reason ever
*   comprehends.*
The lunatic, the lover, and the
*   poet,*
Are of imagination all compact.

—WILLIAM SHAKESPEARE
A MIDSUMMER NIGHT'S DREAM

CHAPTER ONE

Ellen's Story

What follows is essentially the story of a quest, the story of a young woman growing up and attempting to formulate an answer to the question, 'Who am I?' throughout the various phases of her life, and in the varied circumstances in which she found herself, and in which she chose to place herself.

But the chronicle of events in Ellen's life could be interpreted and configured in a radically different manner. In fact it undoubtedly was interpreted in such a manner by the mental health experts who examined Ellen and subjected her to their purportedly scientific scrutiny. In the events and circumstances of the lives of individuals who are psychiatrically labelled the experts see delineated a number of variations on the same essential plot: a mentally damaged individual employs various strategies to sustain the illusion that there is nothing wrong with him or her. It is useful to remember, as the Rosenham study cited below illustrates, that these same kinds of stories were generated by 'experts' about individuals whom they *mistakenly* believed to be 'mental patients'.

The Mental-Health Expert's Approach

The formula that is automatically employed for producing these stories is simple. Firstly: interpret virtually all behavior as psychopathological, as symptomatic. Secondly: explain this symptomatic behavior by portraying it, as Thomas Scheff writes, as "unfolding relentlessly out of a defective psychological system contained within the body". More often than not, today it is asserted to be a defective physiological system, or combination of a defective psychological system and defective physiological system, that accounts for the pathological behavior. If a person is unhappy, for example, that state is assumed to be both a symptom of a damaged psyche and evidence that the person is damaged. All environmental influences are ignored.

In this chapter I will allow the (imaginary) mental health expert to have his or her say, to interrupt our narrative from time to time to tell his or her version. (For the reader's convenience, I have left out a lot of the technical jargon normally used.) I am also making the assumption that our expert's interpretations of Ellen's life were made after her hospitalization and were influenced by his or her awareness of that fact. I'm quite familiar with the mental health experts' procedure for interpreting individuals' lives, since I have a Ph.D. in psychology and I spent many years studying and employing this procedure. When I first began to use it I believed that I was uncovering the real truth, what Freudians call the essential 'psychodynamics' of the individual. I wrote reports similar to that of our expert and received the highest grades. Later, looking back critically, I wrote that these methods for interpreting and assessing individuals

> systematically reduced persons to patients. All of their [the experts'] efforts to understand their 'patients' are guided by a single question: 'What is wrong?' At the end of their investigations (for example 'psychodiagnostic' testing), they present a long list of pathological defects and announce confidently that they have been led inexorably to the conclusion that indeed nothing is right—or at least nothing that has any relevance for the psychotherapist. It is overlooked, of course, that the investigators' questions predetermined the selection and organization of the data. The complexity of a human being, with all his or her manifest or latent talents, dreams and fears, is obscured as therapists persevere at 'scientific' efforts to describe and comprehend a person in terms of a limited set of variables measuring pathology.

Contrasting the two stories will help the reader to grasp the mechanisms by which mental health experts degrade and devalue individuals and impede young people in their efforts to establish a sense of worth and personal identity. In the tale told by the mental health expert, the individual is construed in such a way that his or her life loses all qualities of goal-directedness, of intentionality, of heroism, of grandeur, of mystery, of quest, of meaning. He or she appears in these tales as a pathetic victim of circumstances beyond his or her control, as a being who merits pity but not as a person deserving of respect or reverence.

Spiritual Awakening

I had known Ellen about a year when I had interviewed her. I did not know her very well but already I had been struck by her eloquence, her intelligence, and her perspicacity. She is a creative person who would be described as 'highly functioning' in the words of the mental-health experts; at that time she was working in the advertising department of a women's magazine and had been involved in a romantic relationship with a man for slightly under a year. They recently became engaged to be married. She has returned to college to study education. She is a 28-year-old woman with dark curly hair, assertive yet not aggressive, physically attractive in a striking yet quiet way.

Her story begins during the time of her adolescence, a time when she first became aware of and troubled by the state of the world around her. She describes lonely times and happy times. Her brief tenure at college in 1979 was a time of spiritual awakening, discovery, and challenge. Her retreat from the challenge and her five-year involvement with the mental health system was a harrowing experience for her, "a living Hell on Earth". Later she mused: had she accepted the challenge despite her fears in 1979, she would have been spared a great deal of pain. Unwittingly, the moves she made in 1979 resulted in her accepting later what was probably a far greater challenge.

When Ellen was 11 or 12 years old she began to experience a change in her life. "I started feeling very, very alone. I started contemplating a lot more, on a philosophical kind of note, feeling very alone and alienated. . . . I was feeling disconnected from the suburban lifestyle and from the life that my parents led. I was seeking something deeper." She had an uncle whom she respected who had been in 'primal therapy' and who encouraged her to look inward, to examine and remember the periods of pain that she had had in her life. "At school I felt my friends were very immature and very girly, and very different from me."

The Expert: As a defense against the pressures of a world that threatened the identity of a self that was defective due undoubtedly to parental deprivation at an early stage of development, the patient became preoccupied with her inner thoughts, she regressed to a primitive level of ideation.

The first 10 years of Ellen's life on the other hand had been very happy. "From my earliest memories through about 10 years old I was very happy, very affectionate, outward but a bit shy, but very much a lover of people, humanity, animals, children—a very integrated kind of a girl, very happy and joyous, at peace and innocent."

The Expert: The characterological defenses lead to the repression of traumatic experiences and to an obviously over-idealized depiction of her childhood. The superficial sense of happiness is undoubtedly a reaction-formation against the underlying sense of emptiness.

Ellen withdrew increasingly from the outside world. "And I just became more involved with my psyche, my mind, my darkness, my feelings of being alienated from my contemporaries. . . . At 12, 13, 14 years I became more inward and less involved with people, real curious about my mind. I would think a lot, I would write a lot of poetry, smoke marijuana, and spend a lot of time within my own world. And feeling very connected with nature—that was always my thread . . ."

The Expert: We can detect here the beginning of a schizophrenic deterioration: an inadequate source of self-esteem is preventing her from establishing satisfying 'object relations' that will enable her to meet the demands of adolescence.

There's no reason to assume that Ellen is a defective human being. She's a highly sensitive young woman who was beginning to ask questions about life. She is alienated from her peers who are more superficial and less reflective than she is. If one takes the context into account, the only kind of 'value-free' statement that can be made with confidence is that there is not a *fit* between Ellen and the environment into which she has been cast. This leads to the subjective experience of estrangement. The expert's inference that Ellen has a weak ego is unwarranted. Unhappiness is not a conclusive indication of 'psychopathology'.

Ellen would ask herself, 'What are we here for? What are we doing? You know, what's it all about? How are we going to give each other humanity, and make the world a better place?' Ellen speaks here with the voice of the social critic: "And I knew there must be something more to life than this boring existence that my family led. Also my family was, my mother is very much, you know, concerned about etiquette and properness and what-will-the-neighbors-think."

It is the fate of artists, visionaries, heretics, individuals who are in some ways ahead of their time, to experience alienation. This inability or refusal to reconcile oneself to the *status quo* is a mark of the individual who is destined to change the world in some way. Individuals who are content with the *status quo* have no motivation to work for change. It is creative discontent that is the motor of social evolution.

During her adolescence Ellen was looking around her and making a critique of the values and norms of the culture. This girl, who would later be 'diagnosed' as a 'manic-depressive', was making observations about society similar to those made by various social critics including the *psychiatrist* R.D. Laing, who had written, "Social adaptation to a dysfunctional society may be very dangerous." And: "The condition of alienation, of being asleep, of being out of one's mind, is the condition of the normal man."

She observed with dread the spiritual vacuity of institutional religion as represented by her parents:

> My parents were Catholic. I have one sibling, a brother, two years older. And he and I were pushed into going to church all our lives, and Catholic Sunday School, and to our confirmation. And when we ever asked, why, what is it about, what's the point? I mean, we never felt inspired. I never felt an inspiration from Catholicism or from Christianity as I knew it. It was just boring and bland and you felt—you know, we were doing it because our parents wanted us to do it. And yet, when we asked, why, what is your belief, what's the love, where is it, they really had nothing to offer. It was really that they wanted to do that because they were made to do it, and it was something that they needed to live out, out of their own guilt. And, the fact that we were asking them questions that they really couldn't ask themselves created a bit of a problem, because they were not able to touch, in their own self, what I was bringing out, what I was suggesting to them. They saw in us questions that arose that they were unable to really come to terms with. And so they put the power trip, you know, 'We're your parents; this is what we say; therefore you do it.' Rather than really getting down to the dirt and explaining. And that never sat well with me. I was always a person who asked why. You know, why do we have to do this, why is that the way it is. And their answers never really satisfied me. So I felt a sense of imprisonment, and my own originality, my personality, my desires were coming more

strongly through, and the sense of conviction to my beliefs, even though I wasn't clear about my belief system. I mean, it was just beginning. I was just beginning to check things out and see that the world isn't, you know, The Jones Family and that's it.

Her teens continued to be in general a lonely period for Ellen. She felt very depressed: "I think mainly the root of that was because I wasn't getting support from anywhere." She disliked the 'competitiveness' in her school.

I just didn't want to go to a public school. There were a lot of students, people that I just did not feel connected with. And I was much more artistic, and I used to do a lot of pottery, and I would write poetry, and I was involved with things that I wasn't really allowed to explore in a typical mainstream education. And there was no one to share this with, no one on my wavelength. And I remember reading *Summerhill* and wishing I could go to England. I felt like I was born in a century that I didn't belong in.

The Expert: We can detect here the signs of the patient's incipient psychosis. Due to the fragility of her ego she was not able to enter into normal relationships with her peers, they appear to threaten the precarious sense of stability she had achieved. She rationalizes this inability by assuming an attitude of superiority to her peers. She seeks compensation for the impoverishment of her interpersonal life by retreating into a dream world.

Estranged from the individuals in her environment, from the shallowness, the competitiveness, the hypocrisy of the world around her, like Thoreau Ellen turns to nature. "I was very much in love with nature and, you know, the mountains and animals and lakes and ocean, and that's where I would find refuge from all this horror around me."

In tenth grade Ellen changed schools. She went to a private school and this produced a dramatic change in her life: "I loved it. It was a very artistic, earthy kind of place, with people that were very much like me."

Of course, this fact substantiates the idea that Ellen was unhappy not because she had a defective psychological system but because she had not found a *fit* with her environment. The expert would overlook this datum in his report or declare that Ellen exaggerated her sense of satisfaction.

> So, it was a lovely year. I did a lot with clay, I met some wonderful friends, I loved being up in the mountains and with horses and with lovely trails and nature—I mean, I had a great time. And then after that year I learned of an alternative school in Westchester that was very much geared toward the Outward Bound philosophy of using nature to really push one's own limited perspective of their capabilities and abilities, to really stretch oneself and learn. And that was great. And after that I went away to college in Vermont, Goddard College, a very experimental, very self-motivating kind of a place.

Mystical Experiences

After finishing high school Ellen decided to continue her education at Goddard, an experimental college where the students are given a high degree of freedom to design their own course of study. There is little emphasis on grading or testing. The intellectual standards are rigorous but the students and faculty tend to be unconventional; in another time they would be described as being part of the 'counter-culture'.

The boarding school Ellen had gone to was small, intimate. She had felt a sense of belonging. Goddard immediately struck her as different. It did not have the structure that the boarding school had. It was exciting but it was also a bit frightening at first "and here was this great big pasture to play in and explore myself, with all the freedom I could ever wish for. And I think it was a bit too much for me." She felt she lacked the internal discipline that would have enabled her to fully take advantage of what the school offered. "It was too unstructured."

It was an exciting time as well as a stressful time. Ellen was involved with her studies and inspired by the natural beauty of the countryside and she had a number of ecstatic and spiritual experiences as well as the unpleasant experience of feeling out of place and inadequate. There were many people there that she felt were more mature and defined than she herself was. "There were very fierce individualists there . . . real hard drivers, people who knew what they wanted artistically, politically, socially." They were 'socially minded young adults' who wanted to 'make waves' and change the world. "There was a lot more maturity in these individuals than I had in terms of enduring this kind of free-floating space at Goddard."

The Expert: Due to the impairment of her psyche the patient is unable to adjust to her environment. She projects her internal sense of chaos onto the world in an attempt to avoid coming to terms with her pathology.

Ellen felt that most of the people there had a sense of ethnic identity and groundedness in place that she lacked. Although this made Ellen insecure she also seemed aware of the positive aspects of her relative detachment from place: a heightened sense of universalism, of openness to a variety of peoples.

> My sense of perspective was a bit broader, universal. I think . . . I never felt that I came from a certain shelf on a table or door or country or political slant, religious slant. I felt as if I was a flower in a meadow with lots of other flowers. I mean, I never felt I am Ellen Jones, I'm a girl, I'm from a Catholic background, I'm from New York. I had a different sense of universalness . . . a lack of division among different people for color, religion, age. As a young girl, I think I mentioned to you, and through my life I've had friends that were little babies and 90-year-old women and men.

Although Ellen did not feel clearly defined and grounded she did not lack words or metaphors to describe the sense of identity that she *did* have, as we saw in the preceding paragraph. These metaphors were not the exudate of a defective psychological system. They proved that her self-concept was not totally without content. She was essentially a *seeker.* She may not have had *answers* but she had *questions* and from her words and her demeanor as I interviewed her I knew that even in the midst of self-doubt and distress she appreciated the dignity and purpose of the quest. "I was still just shaping and climbing and, you know, my great attachment was working with clay, and I had visions of working with my art that, more from a fantasy point of view than a reality. . . . I was very vague and yet wanted to explore. I was checking out this, checking out that."

We cannot understand Ellen's experience if we abstract it from the context of her environment. Once again she did not quite fit in, and this generated a sense of internal unease. Whereas in public school she felt more reflective and aware than her peers, at Goddard she felt less developed and this brought up feelings of inadequacy. "It was the individual's sense of character and strength, and the absolute passion within the soul, like burning artists ready to paint, that I didn't feel I had. . . . All of a sudden I didn't feel I measured up so much with the others. I didn't feel as strong individually."

There were other factors that undoubtedly contributed greatly to Ellen's sense of insecurity. She did not get along with her room-mate who would always bring different men home with her. She felt no compunction about having sexual relations with these men while Ellen was in her bed a few feet away. "There was a feeling of not really having a space of my own to come home to every night."

Despite Ellen's anxiety and self-doubts she had several experiences at Goddard those few months that left a mark on her soul, that influenced profoundly the orientation towards life that she was gradually developing. It was these experiences ultimately that *saved* Ellen: that gave her the confidence in her own uniqueness and mission that undergirded her through the times of her greatest self-doubt, and fear. They gave her the strength not to succumb to the experts' diminished view of who she was and who she could become, not to surrender completely when the mental health establishment launched its brutal attack on her sense of self-esteem. These experiences imbued her with the faith that enabled her finally to escape from the clutch of the mental health establishment and complete the journey home to herself, as she put it.

Ellen described her few months at Goddard as a time of "spiritual awakening". "I felt very heightened and got some messages, very powerful kinds of spiritual messages." I asked her to elaborate.

A lot of that was due to being in nature. . . . Just the physical geography of the space was so beautiful and breathtaking. And that was a part of everybody else's souls there. We were all really affected by the stars and the air, and there was a certain magicalness to this section of Vermont, and I found that about Vermont. You know, as soon as you cross the Massachusetts border, you can see and feel you're in Vermont. There is something heavy there and, even with other students that I talked with about that, there was a very mystical sense and, as if it had been, you know, maybe way back a ritual space for American Indians, or something. There was something really in the earth there. I remember walking down the road one night and I had recently read one of Carlos Castañeda's books. And I remember seeing—I don't even remember the book, and it's too bad. But I can remember the memory, this vision of walking down the road and seeing this little thing on the road, like, something just popped there from nowhere.

I asked her if she thought it was an elf.

Yeah—not really an elf, but it was some kind of, some kind of a little magical creature, like, a little magical creature that was somehow described in this Castañeda book I had recently read. And it blew my mind. I just stood there looking at this, and then it disappeared just as it had come. And I remember being on that, you know, on that edge of thinking, 'Am I hallucinating this?' And I knew it was real, and it was just so fascinating to me that I could open up that much to see something like that. It was a very powerful experience to think of breaking down a lot of my own barriers, and my vision opening to outer bounds. I mean, coming in, taking in threads of all kinds of awakenings. Do you know what I'm saying?

I remarked that these kinds of experiences have been exiled from the modern computerized world.

The Expert: The characterological defenses that the patient used to maintain her weak hold on reality have broken down. She is unable now to distinguish between fantasy and reality. We can see that the psychopathology is deep-seated and we can predict that a schizophrenic breakdown is imminent. This is a tragic case, the prognosis is poor.

Ellen recollected another peak experience, to borrow Abraham Maslow's phrase.

And I can remember one time being outside on the deck of this dorm, being outside alone, and the stars were so bright. You ever notice sometimes when you're at the ocean and just breathing in the smell and sound, and you're so soothed and uplifted? . . . And this was one of those moments of being outside, and just opening and easy and loving life so much. That kind of brilliancy that comes through, where you feel like, 'Ahh, this is what it's all about.' Do you know what I mean about the special moments? It's like almost an astrological lining up. You know, how they talk about different planets as if they are all lined up. I mean, there are moments in our lives that we are in such a straight line, the Kundalini energy shoots straight up the spine to one's crown or the chakras are all open. I mean, I don't have a real philosophy, you know, a determining statement. But there are those moments that the sensation is just so powerful, like, 'This is what life is. This is the space I love reaching.'

I responded, "I am thinking of experiences I've had where it's like breaking through the seams of what we take to be reality and then just being aware that one *exists,* that one *is."*

"Yes, that's exactly what it felt like, like you shaved down the mind, you shaved down the body. I mean, it's like all those other things become backdrops and you're with your essence."

I responded, "It's like experiencing existence. Heidegger said, 'This is the age of the forgetfulness of Being'. And all of a sudden it's illuminated, it's there, one's aware that one exists. . . . You know, that's the beginning."

"Yes, yes, it's quite a profound experience, it comes infrequently for me."

The Expert: Unable to deal with responsibilities of the real world, the patient escapes into a fantasy world of her own creation. The schizophrenic deterioration continues inexorably.

As I turned the tape over I mentioned to Ellen that I had been studying a number of Christian thinkers and that they took quite seriously, as did Jesus, the idea of salvation.

Ellen responded by recounting another experience she had had at Goddard.

I never believed in Jesus Christ. . . . I mean, the Catholic background was just kind of, you know, like a hall we were supposed to walk down every Sunday. . . . And, in fact, I didn't even believe in Jesus being a person that had lived or an entity. And it was more through an art history class I had taken that so much art was focused around this so-called individual. And I told the other students that I didn't believe it. I bring that up only because at this one point, that night I was standing on the deck, I remember feeling this energy, this kind of voice from Jesus Christ. And it was bizarre because I didn't believe in this entity, I didn't have any connection with him. I felt him bringing a message to me, as if I was something on Earth like a messenger or a servant—not a servant, but that I had something to say in my lifetime. And I mean, it sounds so tacky, and

I've heard people say this before, like 'Jesus spoke to me last night', you know. And it sounds real hokey and I don't think I ever brought it up because it sounds so hokey, and it's hard to believe that really happened. But I remember feeling so inspired—just like believing in my life a little bit differently from a spiritual sense. And it didn't really matter where that message came from, if it was Buddha or whoever. But it felt to me at that point that it was Jesus talking to me saying, 'Hey, you know, you can do something beautiful on this Earth', or 'Stick to your guns', or something like that.

I asked her if it was actual words that she had heard.

It was like a message through my mind in words . . . it was a phrase. . . . It came from outside through me. . . . I don't remember the exact words, just the feeling of being a very unique individual on Earth, that I had something to give, something to show, something to say. And it was encouraging to know that no matter how much combat you're going to run into, that's what life is like for you, and it's OK.

The Expert: The patient has all the symptoms of a schizophrenic disorder. We detect the pathology in full bloom. She is plagued by auditory hallucinations, magical thinking characteristic of the person who has regressed to a primitive (infantile) level of development. There are grandiose religious delusions. The grandiosity is a compensation for the feelings of inadequacy resulting from damage done to the psyche at an early stage of her development. She should be placed under psychiatric care immediately and put on a strict regimen of medication. Due to the severity of the pathology the patient will need to remain on medication for the rest of her life. Overstimulation ought to be avoided as it may reactivate the schizophrenic disorder.

Retreat and Crisis

I mentioned to Ellen that the typical therapist would regard these experiences as signs of illness. "Yes, I know. And that's one of the reasons I didn't bring it up in therapy. I knew it would be put against me as another note in my documented case." It is not my intention here to *interpret* these experiences. I am aware that mental-health experts would regard her claim to being a 'messenger' as pathological and grandiose. From my viewpoint it constitutes a *leadership claim* that is *validated* by the story told here.

Ellen stayed at Goddard for several months. The tensions with her room-mate continued, her sense of self-esteem remained shaky. "Finally I got to this point where I realized I couldn't really stay afloat in that environment and all the panic buttons went off. I left school. I went back to my parents' house."

Her father came up to get her. She thought to herself, "I don't know what's wrong, I don't know, but this is not right for me now. I'm not able to study. I can't function well. I have to leave and come back to it some other time.... And I felt very ashamed, internally, of having to let go of an experience that I might find something far out in, which is why I came to that school to begin with."

The way Ellen sees it retrospectively is that she copped out. She lacked 'the courage of her convictions'. If she had stayed at Goddard and persevered in spite of her anxieties it would ultimately have been easier than the path she did take, a long painful detour through mental hospitals and day-treatment centers before she finally asserted her independence. Retrospectively she thought to herself: if there had been some support at the time she might have stayed at Goddard and resolved her identity crisis, as she finally did a number of years later.

Ellen did not have anyone to talk to who could understand her situation and she lacked the one resource that might have enabled her to retain her sense of self-integrity through her phase of searching: a room of her own. This fact ought not to be underestimated. Wandering through unfamiliar territory, awed and inspired by her discoveries, fascinated yet intimidated by the powerful individuals she met, she had no familiar terrain where she could retreat and "recollect in tranquility" her experience. She was experiencing the plight of the exile.

She returned to her parents' home. "I came back to this environment that was so totally, you know, submissive and tight and clenching my spirit. I mean, that whole neighborhood and the people I grew up with and the lack of intellectual social stimulation. It was a very narrow-minded sort of country town that I had grown up in."

She felt disappointed in herself, frustrated, she would get angry a lot often for seemingly trivial reasons. "I'd drive the car, and if a guy ahead of me didn't go through the green light quickly enough I would get nuts and bang on the steering wheel and beep."

She had left Goddard in November of 1979. It was now autumn of 1980. Some of her anger was directed at her father and her brother who she felt were over-controlling. "My anger frightened me. All of a sudden anger came out of nowhere. Perhaps it was because I never learned to express it and it would build up and I'd fly off the handle."

That fall Ellen was involved in an automobile accident (she was not at fault). The injuries were minor but the experience was traumatizing. After the accident she had trouble eating and was anxious a lot of the time. "My parents were worried. And *that* frightened me to see their fear. So it was kind of a thing that was crescendoing." She went to see a therapist (a social worker) who kept trying to persuade her to go to a mental hospital to get some 'rest' and 'privacy' and 'nurturing'. Finally she agreed on Christmas Eve day to go see a psychiatrist.

The Mental Hospital

The psychiatrist informed her she was having a nervous breakdown and said it was imperative that she be hospitalized as soon as possible. She was hospitalized and immediately put on 'medication': Thorazine and Navane.

Ellen described the effects of these toxic psychiatric drugs. "I lost my sense of vision. I couldn't read." She said that it would not be accurate to describe the effects of the drugs as 'tranquilizing'. "It was heavy sedation. I slept about three days straight." When she woke up they continued to give her drugs. "They made me feel totally numbed out, catatonic, totally apathetic."

Her vision remained blurred. "My dad took me to an eye doctor while I was in the hospital, thinking it was a physical thing, but the eye doctor said, 'Oh no, it's the Thorazine, that's the effect it has on the eyes.'"

She was frightened that her vision was blurred. "The doctors took me off Thorazine and put me on Navane and Lithium as well." Her vision cleared up. However, the drugs continued to have a deleterious effect on her mind and body.

> I was about 120 pounds when I entered. And, you know, within five or six months I was about 50, 60 pounds heavier. I was

walking the halls and my body was barely able to move. There was no fluidity to my movement. I was this big, stiff, massive thing. And it was like all this physical sensation and nothing spiritual, no light, no beauty.

This dramatic change in Ellen's physical form struck at the very core of her sense of femininity. "There was a lot of self-doubt. The fact that my body was so different, it was so distorted, I was so fat, I was 20, 21 years old." She got out of the hospital and continued taking the drugs: "I would hide, I would wear big, loose things without showing my body. I wouldn't swim."

She felt estranged from her natural body rhythms. "I was shut down totally. I was constipated, I had a dry mouth. I gained 80 pounds in the whole period. Hormonally everything changed. My whole body totally shifted. Every little cell was different, beating on a different note. And I really lost touch with my true essence. I felt like a dead person in a body that lived."

Ellen's experience is typical. The majority of people whom I have talked to have found these drugs very unpleasant at best. Ellen, like many other patients, stopped taking the drugs. "I would slip it under my tongue and spit it out. And my parents saw that once, and they called the doctors, so I had to have liquid medication to drink in front of them."

The Expert: This is a treatment-resistant patient. She overlooks the beneficial features of the medication and focuses exclusively on its unpleasant but comparatively insignificant side-effects. Unable to acknowledge that her sense of disorientation is an effect of her psychopathology, she claims that it is purely an effect of the medication.

The psychiatrist told Ellen that she had a combination of a number of different mental illnesses. "He didn't know what to put his finger on." Later he decided she was a 'manic-depressive'. Ellen was astute enough to capture the gist of what was being conveyed to her. "I was not OK, not right, not healthy, not correct."

Szasz has written:

the vocabulary of psychiatric diagnoses is in fact a massive pseudomedical justificatory rhetoric of rejection. In short,

psychiatrists are the manufacturers of medical stigma, and
mental hospitals are their factories for mass-producing this
product. . . . Being considered or labeled mentally disordered
—abnormal, crazy, mad, psychotic, sick, it matters not what—
is the most profoundly discrediting classification that can be
imposed on a person today. Mental illness casts the 'patient'
out our social order just as surely as heresy cast the 'witch' out
of medieval society.

When Ellen was taken to the hospital she was at first partly
relieved to be told she was mentally ill.

I didn't really, truly, internally believe what they were saying
about me, but yet, in a rational sense, there was part of
me . . . that was relieved that there was such a diagnosis, such
descriptions, so that I finally fit into something. . . . finally
fitting into a mold, into a classification, even though it was a
pathological one, and a disease-oriented one. . . . But that was
very short-lived.

On the one hand the tension of Ellen's identity crisis—Who
am I?—was attenuated. She was no longer living suspended over
an abyss of uncertainty. On the other hand at the cost of her
dignity she could gain all the benefits of the sick role, the benefits
of dependency, of being defined as a helpless incompetent and
taken care of.

Ellen astutely described the process whereby individuals
become inducted into the role of chronic mental patients.

People sold out for acceptance, whether it's the acceptance of
being a good manic-depressive or a good schizophrenic or
whatever. . . . I think that some people were so unsure of who
they were, they were without any sense of definition. And when
they came into this very freaked-out, emotional state—a lot of
fear, and here are, like, these big authorities saying, 'Oh, it's
OK, this is where you belong. This is what we're going to do for
you.' People really surrendered, and I just didn't.

Although—Ellen added—many of the friends she made in
mental hospitals could not bear the loss of dignity and seeing no
alternative way out, they killed themselves.

Although Ellen did not surrender—on the deepest level of her
soul she refused to define herself as a mentally damaged person
—in order to get out of the mental hospital she acted out the role
expected of her. "I played a game to get by. It wasn't even a game,
it was survival. . . . I knew that the only way to get through the
ropes was to kind of play along with the game, or else they'd send

me to a state mental hospital, and I might be committed for life."
There is no 'paranoia' in Ellen's testimony: in the mental health
system anything less than total compliance is viewed as a threat.
Any criticism of the mental health system is viewed as a sign of
'serious psychopathology'. This is documented not only by my
interviews with patients and therapists but also by research
studies. Consequently, in order to have any chance of escaping
from the system, one has to confirm the definition given to one
by one's captors: one must acknowledge that one is a mentally
defective individual in need of psychiatric help and guidance.

Ellen's compliance was not a consciously deliberated strategy.

> Part of it was conscious and part of it was not. Part of me
> sensed that I was not really a mental defective but that I had to
> protect myself by going along with the game. And another part
> of me knew, or I should say suspected, that the good manic-
> depressive I pretended to be was not who I really was, and
> sensed that at some point I'd get salvation.

Ellen observed and became aware of the limitations of the
professionals, the ways in which their own fears prevented them
from being helpful.

> Sometimes you ask people questions that are unresolved
> within themselves. And they are not able in their own lives to
> look at it and face it. So they want to quiet you down. I felt that
> way with psychiatrists and social workers and, you know, the
> whole AMA at large, that one of the reasons why they're so
> quick to diagnose and shelve and label somebody and treat
> them in a certain way is because they're frightened by seeing
> someone else's inquisitiveness and ability to touch their own
> bare souls and pain and suffering. And instead of responding to
> that within themselves, it's, you know, the power trip and the
> ego and the ability to quiet someone with drugs or with a silent
> room or with no passes or whatever. It's a way that they don't
> have to ever touch that. But they can stay continually detached,
> and get society's respect by being a psychiatrist or whatever.

Her awareness, her ability to see through the facade, helped
her survive her mental hospital experience. "It helped me stay
alive . . . it kept me somewhat sane, shall we say." I asked her
what gave her such confidence in her own perceptions and vision.
"I have no idea. I think there is a definite spiritual bent to me,
that I have a fire, that I'm supposed to be flaming in this life. I
don't know. I am just strong-willed and when I see something
that's true, I don't renege. I won't let go."

The Day Hospital

Part of the process of being inducted into a career as a chronic
mental patient is to attend a 'day hospital' or a 'day treatment'
program after one is released from the mental hospital. Usually
the pretense is made that this a stepping-stone back into society.
In actual fact it securely seals one's permanent exile from the
'normal' world. All of the procedures impress upon the individual that he or she is different and defective. The total lack of any
opportunity to engage in the kind of meaningful work that
typically earns one esteem in this society guarantees that the
individual will be cut off from the kind of input that could
potentially restore her self-respect. In the name of mental health,
billions of individuals have had their dreams destroyed in these
ostensibly therapeutic institutions. Ellen survived.

"I was there for a number of months. It was horribly depressing because you're with people that are half-dead, three-quarters-
dead. You just felt as if you were in a big cow herd, with one
cowboy pushing you down. It was awful."

The social workers there would give them daily lessons on how
to groom and take care of themselves. Ellen remarked, "As if we
did not know how to brush our own hair. As if I was totally
incapable of taking care of myself. And this is very, very
embarrassing for individuals at that vulnerable stage of their life
development."

The Expert: Most of the individuals are so incapacitated by
their illnesses that they have forgotten how
to do the kinds of activities that are routine
for most of us. Like many individuals afflicted with mental illnesses Ellen chooses to
suppress the memory of how debilitated she
was.

It was like being in grade school again. "You have to have a
van come to your house and pick you up and drive you to this day
hospital to be with people that are *so* numbed out and dead and
manipulated. And actually some of my dearest friends through
those years had taken their own lives. And some were so totally,
overly drugged that they had no sense of their genuine qualities
or their light."

The consumption of psychiatric drugs is detrimental in a
number of ways. Not only does it adversely affect the body and

mind but the daily consumption of these drugs ('medication') constitutes a ritual of degradation reminding one that one is not like normal people. "The message is, 'You're messed up. You're sick. You're not OK to live in society without taking a prescription remedy.'" She kept asking the psychiatrists to take her off the drugs: "'Come on. I don't want to do it. What's the point? I don't want it.' And he would always threaten me. 'Oh, no, if you stop taking the drugs you'd go nuts.'" Ellen's experience is typical.

The Expert: The patient refuses to accept the fact that she is a manic-depressive and will inevitably decompensate [the fragile defenses that protect her 'defective' psyche will stop functioning] if she discontinues the medication for any length of time. She denies her pathology and claims her low self-esteem is a result of having to take medication.

Ellen found the staff was invariably patronizing. "They act as if you are pathetic, like they feel sorry for you, as if you're doomed to spend the rest of your life there because you're not competent to do anything else. And it's a struggle to maintain your dignity when you're surrounded by people who let you know in subtle and not so subtle ways that they regard you as a loser."

Getting Out of the System

Jay Haley has argued that the longer a young person is involved with the mental health system the more difficult it is to reintegrate him or her into society.

The family and community organize around the young person as an invalid, which makes the therapist's work more difficult. The longer he or she is in custody or treatment, the more the young person settles into the career of a mental patient, not only within the family but also with the deviants he associates with in treatment settings. . . . The prophecy of social controllers that a person is handicapped and must remain in custody or on medication for life is often fulfilled by the 'treatment' which socially handicaps the person for life.

Ellen was in danger of becoming a professional mental patient.

She was becoming increasingly dissatisfied with the system. The mental health experts made no effort to encourage her to wean herself from Lithium. They failed to convey to her confidence in her ability to handle the challenges that would be involved in the kind of life to which she truly aspired. "I was living with my parents, all my other friends were graduating and going to law school or medical school, or artists, or whatever. And here I was this big round ball without any definition in her own mind. All my dreams, all my fantasies, all the things that had kept me alive, all disappeared. My sense of vision deteriorated."

In 1984 she decided to get off Lithium. "After many years of taking it I just realized that it was poison, as if I was polluting myself, hurting myself, killing myself with these drugs." "I needed to stand strong for who I was beyond everybody else's fear."

In October 1984 Ellen went to Massachusetts to live with an old boyfriend. She discontinued taking Lithium. At first all went smoothly but he then became abusive and they had frequent conflicts. She felt under great stress and was having trouble sleeping. In January 1985 she returned to the hospital in New York, thinking maybe the authorities were right about her.

At the end of the year she dropped out of the day treatment center, stopped seeing her therapist, and got a job as a file clerk. Her therapist felt that it was a mistake to terminate therapy and that she was not ready to work. But she was determined now finally to achieve independence.

In the beginning of 1987 she had saved up enough money and found an apartment in New York City. She worked as a secretary to a chiropractor. Over a four-month period she decreased the Lithium until she was completely free of it. She told no one at the time about this since she anticipated that their fearful reactions might have an adverse effect on her.

What explained Ellen's sudden resolve? "The spiritual sense was growing so strong that it kind of shot through the rest and said, 'I won't let this happen to you. I'm going to take care of you, I'm not going to let your mind and body be destroyed by jerks out there.'"

It's strange that I waited that long—until the stakes were at their highest, when my body was used to years of psychiatric drugs, when it was the most dangerous time, in a way, because if I faltered who knows if I would have survived. *It was as if my soul waited for the most powerful—I mean, I was restricted to the most confining space you can be, besides being gagged and tied.* I mean, to be chemically induced for so long. To stop that and say, 'No. It's my time to free myself and really live in the way I choose to.' And one aspect of it—I mean, in one way it was the easiest time because the situation was so severe that there was no other choice. In my heart there was no other choice. But on the other hand, it would have been easier, looking back in sort of a hypothetical situation, it would have been easier at Goddard, at that point, to go on, before I had years of psychiatric history and stigma and drugs. But it was as if my own awakening took place at, you know, a very crucial forkroad. Do you know what I mean?

I responded, "Yes."

And it's interesting to see that how that rebirthing is so much more powerful and integrated when there's so much against you. It's like a concentration camp inmate just fleeing—when the thing got so bad that it would be better to be shot in the field than live like that. You know, you have to break free, affirm your spirit, and try. In a way that's what it was like.

She was independent. She had her own apartment. She was working full-time now as a secretary for a chiropractor.

When I got off the Lithium I had the sensation of being home again. It all clicked and it made sense that, 'Oh, I see, I was saving myself for that moment where I would break free and rejoice with myself.' Part of me thought I'd never become independent. So it was a very spiritual, integrated experience of relief, joy, pride, courage. You know, a real sense of coming home and feeling myself for the first time in many years. I had finally claimed myself again in the fertile ground of my being.

The Expert: The diagnosis is manic-depression in remission. The patient's personality disorder prevents her from acknowledging her pathology.

Recapitulation

The first ten years of Ellen's life had been relatively harmonious. She evidently felt a sense of belonging in her family. Ellen was a precocious girl and at about age ten her inner character began to emerge. This resulted in an increasing sense of estrangement as

she became disturbed by the hypocrisy and mindless convention-
ality of her family and of the society around her. She read the
work of visionaries and social critics—she specifically mentioned A. S. Neill and Thoreau. To interpret her sense of
alienation as a symptom of pathology is to define 'mental health'
as acceptance of the *status quo.*

To the sensitive soul, waking up in the universe can be an
excruciatingly painful experience. When the young Siddhartha
(who was to become the Buddha) emerged as a young man from
his cocoon of wealth and family security he was so jolted by the
magnitude of human suffering and the indifference of those who
had seemingly achieved a degree of comfort that he gave up
everything—wealth, security, family—and began his quest. To
the mental health expert this would undoubtedly be interpreted
as a sign that the Buddha's psyche was defective. Henry Miller
wrote, "If we were truly awake we would be stunned by the
horror of our everyday life. No one in his right senses could
possibly do the crazy things which are now demanded of us every
moment of the day." An individual who awakes to the horror,
who wants to change the world, would inevitably feel a sense of
mission, a calling, as it were, to lead his fellow human beings
forward. This is invariably interpreted by the mental health
experts today as a sign that he or she is 'grandiose'. His or her
leadership claim is invalidated by the guardians of the *status quo,*
by the 'mind police'—to borrow Laing's phrase.

Ellen had disembarked. She had left the cloistered world of
her family and was confronted with the task of defining an
identity, of assuming an orientation toward the world that felt
authentic to her, an expression of her inner being. Like the
Buddha, she could not turn back. She could not return to the safe
haven of her family. If she was to find peace, she must seek port
in a new harbor.

Ellen's sense of estrangement was assuaged when she went to
another school and found herself with a group of people similar
to herself. She felt comfortable, inspired, accepted, a sense of
belonging. But this was only a brief respite, a temporary refuge
from the demands of the world.

College faced her with the task of defining her identity. She
met others who were prepared to be leaders, to go out and
'change the world'. Was she adequate to the task? Could she
'measure up'? Ellen was plunged into a crisis. Laing had said that
the role of the therapist is to act as a guide. Ellen found no guides.
She found only pseudo-guides who attempted to place the seal of

Authority, of Medicine, on her exile from herself and from the world.

In pre-modern societies crises were regarded as integral to the process of growth and transformation. The anthropologist Victor Turner describes this as a "liminal" phase: "Here the cognitive schemata that give sense and order to everyday life no longer apply but are, as it were, suspended."[1] This is the precondition for a death-rebirth experience. Turner argues that rites of passages were incorporated into pre-modern cultures to enable individuals to transverse these liminal phases. "Only in this way, through destruction and reconstruction, that is transformation, may an authentic re-ordering come about."[2]

The density of everyday life is ignored in the stories written by the mental health experts. It is always the same monotonous story, of pathological behavior emerging relentlessly out of a defective psychological or physiological system. Liminal phases, growth crises, are seen only as symptoms of pathology. The individual's quest for a sense of personal identity is not recognized. All environmental influences are ignored. The contingent, the seemingly accidental, have no place in these stories. For example, it is reasonable to propose that had Ellen had a space of her own at Goddard she might have had the strength to withstand the process of destruction and reconstruction without fleeing back to her parental home.

In a society that lacks rites of passage the role of the therapist becomes critical. He or she can help the person tolerate the process of change and transformation. He or she can help the young person to confront the unknown, to accept the challenge of leaving home, both in the literal sense of achieving independence from his family of origin, as Haley argues, and in the spiritual sense, as Laing has urged, of rejecting the moribund traditions of a materialist society and affirming the integrity of one's own vision.

Ellen went to the mental health establishment for guidance but discovered that its officers had no interest in encouraging her autonomy. They attempted to induct her into the role of a chronic mental patient. They attempted to solve her identity crisis by conferring on her a degraded social identity.

Szasz writes that the true therapist is a "noble rhetorician

---

[1]Victor Turner, *From Ritual to Theatre* (New York: P.A.J. Publications, 1982), 123
[2]Ibid., 124

[who] uses language to wean men from their inclination to depend on authority, to encourage them to think and speak clearly, and to teach them to be their own masters."[3]

Bruce Wilshire had written that "language is a vehicle for the transformation of self. . . . Metaphors and their entailments may serve to re-organize entire world-views in the process of giving meaning to the self."[4]

The core metaphors of the mental health experts deplete the self of meaning. 'Manic-depressive', 'schizophrenic', 'genetic defect', 'chronic mental illness': these become the metaphors offered to individuals as the key to defining who they are, these become the metaphors that mediate the experience of the self. The mental health establishment has criticized authors such as Laing for 'romanticizing mental illness'. The colonization of the language by medical metaphors has de-romanticized virtually all aspects of human existence, and left the individual stranded in a world bereft of meaning and mystery. Ellen finally realized that this was not the way home—that the mental health experts specialized in the expropriation of the self.

She described breaking away from the mental health system as coming home. "You know, a real sense of coming home and feeling myself for the first time in many years." She gave up the role of the mental patient. She cast aside the metaphors they offered her as clues to the meaning of her self. The woman who had been "vague" and "exploring" at Goddard, who had felt she lacked the passion of many of the other students, now said, "I have a fire . . . I'm supposed to be flaming in this life." Ellen felt she had gone through "this living Hell on Earth for a very meaningful purpose, to be able to touch people and hear their pain and to help them get through it."

[3]Thomas Szasz, *The Myth of Psychotherapy* (New York: Syracuse University Press, 1988), 20

[4]Bruce Wilshire, 'Language and the Self', *Symbolic Interactionism,* 16 (1983), 302

CHAPTER TWO

Kristin's Story

Kristin is a 34-year-old woman. She is a survivor of several psychiatric incarcerations. She has been a psychotherapist for several years. She completed her master's degree in counseling in 1988. She has not been in a mental hospital in seven years. She does not take psychiatric drugs. Throughout her hospitalizations she has consistently refused to take neuroleptic drugs. She took antidepressants for two years in her early twenties. She has been diagnosed as a 'depressive neurotic', a 'pseudo-neurotic schizophrenic', and a 'manic-depressive'.

Kristin's first encounter with the mental health system occurred when she was seven. Her mother thought Kristin was too active and took her to a psychiatrist who diagnosed her as hyperactive. Kristin's sister, who was one year older than her, was physically handicapped and consequently did not move around much. Kristin believed that her mother would have felt more comfortable with a child who "just lay around". "I was just real active, a normal child." The psychiatrist gave her phenobarbital. It had an adverse affect on her. "I remember taking the stuff and running into walls." The administration of the drug was discontinued.

When Kristin was in third grade she had another encounter with the mental health system. Kristin got A's in all her classes except math, where she consistently got D's and F's. An IQ test was administered to her. She did very well on the verbal sub-test and poorly on the performance sub-test. The school psychologist said she had a 'minimal brain dysfunction' that caused a 'learning disability'. No 'remedial' measures were taken at that time.

Home Life

Kristin's childhood and adolescence were not happy. Kristin's mother and father did not have a happy marriage. Her mother drank heavily and her father was in the Air Force so that he was

usually out of town. When he was in town he seemed to have a
closer bonding with Kristin than he did with his wife. Kristin was
his favorite daughter. She thought that her mother was very
critical of her. "No matter what I did, my mother didn't like it."
But the mother was not critical of Kristin's two sisters. Kristin
says that she believes her sisters would corroborate her perception that her mother was more critical of her. When Kristin was a
young adolescent her mother would frequently get drunk and
accuse her of having sex with her father.

Kristin recounts one incident that typifies the pattern that
persisted in her family. "When I was 15 Dad got me a horse. I
loved horseback riding. Shortly afterwards he got himself a horse
and the two of us would go on trips together. I enjoyed this
because I loved my dad and I wasn't getting any attention from
my mother. This made my mother furious, of course, since my
dad was neglecting her."

Throughout Kristin's adolescence a similar sequence of events
would recur continually. Her mother would get drunk and accuse
her of "doing things" with her father. Both she and her mother
would go into their own bedrooms crying. Later her father would
come to her bedroom and say to Kristin, "I know you were right.
It was wrong of your mother to criticize you like that, but I
couldn't say anything. I had to stick by her because she is my
wife."

The situation at school was hardly more felicitous. Kristin's
older sister had skipped three grades, and was in college by age
16. "To keep up with this woman was impossible." The teachers
would constantly say to Kristin, 'You're sure not as smart as your
sister.' Her little sister, who was two years younger, got straight
A's. "I decided to be bad. I started smoking cigarettes, running
around with kids who drank." She never did anything serious
enough to get involved with the police. But she and her friends
would play pranks, such as stuffing the school toilets up with
buns that they had gotten from the cafeteria. Whereas previously
her grades had been satisfactory, now she started getting D's and
F's.

Her mother and her father took her to a psychologist to find
out what was wrong with her. He was an unusual psychologist
who had studied family therapy. After hearing Kristin's story
about her family life he told her that the problem was not in her
but in the way that the family related to each other. He explained
to Kristin that she was 'triangulated': that her parents fought out

their problems through her. He said that he needed to get the family to change. She responded, "Good luck!" He made an appointment for all the family members to come in. When she left his office, she thought to herself, "God, there is actually someone who put into words what I've been feeling for 15 years."

Kristin remembers well the family session. The psychologist was blunt with her parents. "What would you talk about if you didn't have problems with Kristin?" he asked directly. "You need to communicate with each other and to stop putting her in the middle." Kristin's sisters started crying and yelling, "Stop it! Stop it!"

The therapist tried to get Kristin's mother and father to talk to each other about their problems and their conflicts. Her mother got angry and insisted that Kristin had deep emotional problems. Her father was silent but he gave Kristin a look as if to say, "I know he's right but your mother can't take it." Of course she realized that this act was a repetition of the same pattern that the therapist was attempting to change. Her mother led the family members out of the office and said that she was not coming back. Kristin remained. The therapist looked at her and said, "You must convince them to come back."

From a family-therapy perspective—from a systems perspective—this therapist had clearly identified the problem. But he had failed to respond in a competent manner. The therapist's task is not just to correctly identify a problem, but to motivate people to change their behavior. This therapist had attempted to prematurely force a reorganization of the family. As a consequence he alienated them and they walked out. The prominent family therapist Salvador Minuchin would have said that he had challenged the dysfunctional patterns of interaction and assumptions of the family before he had succeeded in 'joining' with them, that is, before he had gained their trust. A family therapist must first gain the trust of all the family members—must be accepted as part of the family—before he can motivate them to change.

Kristin was about 17 at this time. She decided to run away to Florida. "I couldn't stand it any more." She would call her parents from time to time to tell them that she was safe. Her mother threatened to kill Kristin's cat if she did not return. She found some friends in Florida and she survived by panhandling, stealing from grocery stores, and eating turtle eggs, which they would dig up from the sand on the beaches. She explained that this was a good source of protein. She had been reported as a runaway child and the police were looking for her.

Six months after she had left home she was caught by the police and sent home. It was the middle of the year, too late to return to school, so she got a job working in a restaurant. Her two sisters had left home. She was alone with her parents. She was miserable. That summer she stopped working and got her G.E.D.

She considered going to college but at this point her confidence in her intellectual abilities had been shaken. One can easily infer some of the sources of this lack of confidence. Earlier she had been 'diagnosed' as having 'minimal brain dysfunction' and a 'learning disability'. Her triangulation in her parents' marriage was a source of great distress that had a deleterious effect on her performance in school. Her siblings' relative freedom from the marital conflict helped them to excel in school. Her teachers had continually made negative comparisons between her and her sister, further undermining her confidence.

The Expert: The patient's low sense of self-esteem is a result
               of impairment of the ego, suggesting that the
               classical Oedipal neurosis is complicated by
               a narcissistic disorder stemming from early
               childhood. This diagnosis is further corrobo-
               rated by the persistent pattern of rebellion
               and the patient's denial of any pathology.

Marriage and Divorce

She stayed at her parents and went back to work as a waitress. Then a new development occurred. "This guy came along who raced horses and I liked horses, so we ended up getting married." It must have seemed to her as if a golden opportunity had fallen before her: finally an escape from the insufferable conditions at home with her family.

The honeymoon was short-lived. They lived together in a one-room trailer and spent all day working together raising the horses. The constant association caused a lot of tension between them. This was made worse by the fact that he felt threatened when she did a better job training a horse than he did.

One day, approximately six months after the marriage, one of Kristin's girlfriends came down to visit her from a neighboring town. It had been decided before that Kristin and her husband Jack and the girlfriend Sue and a friend of Jack's would go out dancing together. But Jack had been drinking quite heavily that day, something that he infrequently did, and he had passed out on the bed. Kristin said to her girlfriend, "Well, we'll just go out without him." Apparently Jack had awoken and overheard her statement. Almost immediately after she made the suggestion he got up from the bed and walked into the room where they were sitting. He said, "You're going to do what?" Before she had a chance to reply he smacked her a couple of times in the face. He was 6'6" and muscular, she was 5'4" and delicate. At that point she kicked him "in the balls". "He started beating the hell out of me. There was blood everywhere." Kristin's girlfriend was not able to stem the tide of his fury. Finally she ran out of the house crying.

She was taken to the hospital. She had a broken nose. Plastic surgery was performed six months later. She immediately filed for divorce and at his urging dropped the criminal charges against him.

She moved back into her parents' home. "I was emotionally mortified. I love someone enough to marry him and he half kills me. I was paralyzed. I was so stressed out I didn't know what to do. I started hallucinating. Things looked different, as if they were breathing. I went into Mom's bed and was crying. I was seeing colored dots on the wall and I told her about it. I wanted her to hold me and talk to me. I'd always wanted that to happen but I never got it." She tried halfheartedly but it felt awkward. "It didn't feel real."

In the Psychiatric Ward

Her mother begged her to go to the psychiatric ward of the general hospital. She agreed. The psychiatrist in the ward told her that she was suffering from a depressive neurosis. She would meet with him regularly when she was in the hospital. He was a Freudian and he had some unusual ideas. He told her that she was having sex with her father, that she had repressed the memory of it.

He called her father and asked him to come for a session. Dr. Cox said to him, "I know about your incestuous relationship with your daughter."

Kristin's father responded, "I think you have the wrong idea."
Dr. Cox said, "I do not. I will now leave you two alone to talk."

She said neither of them knew what to say. Her father said, "I'm sorry if I haven't been as good a parent as I could have."

He got up to leave the psychiatric ward. Kristin reached up to hug him goodbye. He recoiled. He said, "I'll call you."

Kristin thought, 'Dr. Cox, you asshole. Maybe my dad did triangulate me. But at least he was a parent close to me that I did get some kind of affection from. It's been funny since then. My dad is not that kind of person. He never touched me physically at all.' Dr. Cox had the idea that he would 're-parent' Kristin.

While she was in the hospital she was forced to take antidepressant drugs, which made her nervous. One of her main fears was that she would be 'electro-shocked'. Dr. Cox had told her, "If you do what you're told you will not have to have it." She remembers that Tuesday and Thursday were electro-shock days and Dr. Cox would line everybody up.

> One woman, Frankie, was bummed out because she had walked home one day and found her husband in bed with her best friend. She made a suicide attempt. I don't think it's that abnormal—a reaction to losing the two most important people in your life at once. And Dr. Cox gave her ECT the next day, before the drugs were even out of her system. Then she came back delirious. ECT causes brain damage, which makes you temporarily euphoric. Frankie was giddy and euphoric for a couple of days. She acted silly. But two days later she was sitting right back in the corner, moaning and crying. I would go into the room and try to talk to her. I would say to her, "Do you want to talk?" But the nurses would always come in and say, "Leave her alone. She needs to be alone." Then two or three days later Dr. Cox would come to give her another ECT treatment and she would say, "Oh, no! Not again!"
> I was scared to death they'd give it to me. I thought to myself, 'Don't look depressed, whatever the hell you do. And eat all your supper, for God's sake, and try to think what this 70-year-old man wants you to act like and look like so he doesn't think you are depressed.'

Kristin didn't see anyone who was helped by the ECT. Another woman who had it seemed indifferent when she came back. Kristin noticed that she would just sleep a lot more.

After a month in the hospital Dr. Cox released her. She went home and resumed working as a waitress in a restaurant. She continued to see Dr. Cox once a month for antidepressants and psychotherapy. I asked her why she continued to see him. She said, "The first year and a half I thought he was really going to help. I didn't know what else to do. I thought, 'Maybe he knows something I don't know.' I knew later on, of course, that he didn't. But I thought maybe there was some pill that would make things stop hurting. I know better now."

The sessions did nothing to stimulate her or to boost her self-confidence or to motivate her. "Dr. Cox would ask me questions about my childhood first, and then he would just get bored. Several times he even fell asleep when I was talking. And then he'd just give me another prescription."

The drugs did nothing to make her pain go away. "Why should they?" she asked. "My living situation hadn't changed at all." Her sisters had both escaped from the home and were in college getting all A's. The same pattern persisted in her relationship with her parents. Her mother would get drunk and hit her father, who would sit there passively. She would criticize Kristin viciously. "She told me that she and Dad had a wonderful relationship until I came along." Later in the evening Kristin's father would go to her bedroom and apologize for not sticking up for her. She would ask, "Why didn't you protect me?"

He would start crying and saying, "I just can't."

Sometimes he would go to sleep at the foot of her bed. "He seemed like a lost kid to me. He'd always talk to me about their problems. I felt stuck right in the middle and terrified my mother was going to walk in and hear my father confiding in me."

New Diagnosis, New Drugs

This went on for a year and a half after she got out of the hospital. It was around this time that Dr. Cox decided that she was not a depressive-neurotic after all, but a 'pseudo-neurotic schizophrenic'. He decided to put her on Stelazine and Prolixin. He gave her these new drugs and told her to take them. She agreed.

She went home. "I took the drug and I thought I was going to die. I couldn't walk. I felt a strong disinclination to live. I could not get out of bed. My arms were like metal and the bed was like a magnet. My tongue was all rolled up in my mouth. My toes were in spasms. I couldn't move. I peed in my bed."

The next day she called Dr. Cox and told him that the drugs were making her sick. He said, "I gave you the smallest dosage. It's not possible that you feel that way."

Kristin was shocked. She responded, "But I do! And when I don't take them I don't feel that bad. When I do take them I do."

Dr. Cox responded, "Well, that's just part of your illness. It's a deeper psychosis coming on. I could have predicted this."

"I said to him, 'My eyes were rolling back in my head, my tongue was hanging out of my mouth jerking around and once I could move again I found myself constantly pacing up and down the floor."

Dr. Cox was adamant. "This is part of your illness."

"I said to him, 'Before I went into the hospital all I felt was sad.'"

At this point, her confidence in Dr. Cox was thoroughly undermined. She began to think about things differently. "I felt that I was sad because I had a terrible relationship with my mom and dad, and I went to another relationship that I really depended on and he about half-killed me. I was just very grieved. I was never given the opportunity to grieve. And that's what turned into what they called a 'depression.'"

The next visit that she was scheduled to see him, she got to the office early and snuck into the room where her chart was. It was on the desk. She looked at it. She saw that the diagnosis had been changed from "depressive neurosis" to "pseudo-neurotic schizophrenia". This explained why he had decided to put her on different drugs.

"Were you doing anything differently?" I asked.

She responded that she had started working in a new restaurant and she was dating the grill cook. She thought that Dr. Cox did not approve of her going out with someone with such a lowly occupation, particularly as she herself came from an upper middle-class professional family. Her relationship with the grill cook ended after several months.

By this time she was 24 years old. She'd made friends with Jeff, a man about ten years older than she was and she moved into his three-bedroom house. After living there for several months they became lovers. She felt more confident in herself and she started college.

Her relationship with Jeff was complicated by her parents' opposition. Despite the fact that she was living away from them and had a boyfriend, her parents attempted to include her once again in their relationship. The family would not reorganize to accept Kristin's independence. "I'd call my mom and she said, 'Don't call me, we're not your family any more. Jeff and Timmy are your family now. You have a retarded stepson now to take care of.' " (Jeff's eight-year-old son was slightly retarded.)

Kristin was having a hard time separating from her parents because she had such a strong yearning for their approval. "Jeff was a working-class guy and my parents never approved. I loved him but I was torn. I thought if I got rid of this guy, if I get my college degree, then I'll get approval from my parents. I finally realized that no matter what I did they wouldn't approve."

She remembers vividly one incident that occurred shortly before she and Jeff broke up. Her parents were coming over to visit her and Jeff. Her father called to say that her mother was drunk and had jumped out of the car on the way over. "Please help me find your mother," he pleaded.

Jeff and Kristin got in a car and began to look for her. They found her in a field and brought her back to their home. She started hitting Jeff. "I pulled her off Jeff. She started punching me. She kept hitting me repeatedly, over and over again. Jeff finally succeeded in pulling her off me."

Jeff thought formalizing their relationship might make it stronger. He asked Kristin to marry him. She agreed. He gave her a ring. She was talking to her mother one day on the phone and her mother was criticizing her, saying, "Why do you want to marry him? He's just a factory worker."

She said, "I'm not really engaged to him, I'm going to give him back the ring. I just don't know how to tell him yet."

Jeff heard her. He was very hurt. Two days later he said to her, "When are you going to give back the ring?"

At that point she did not know what to do. She felt torn in different directions. She went out, started getting drunk and sleeping around. On the one hand she felt she loved him, on the other hand she felt that she was "supposed to end up with somebody more educated and more intellectual. I relied on my parents to give him the stamp of approval."

One day she came home from a bar late at night to find that Jeff had taken all her stuff out of the house and loaded it up in her station wagon. She called her mother and went over to her parents' house. She was sleeping on the couch and her mother came out and was "peering" at Kristin. "I started seeing malicious expressions on her face. I thought to myself, 'She's going to kill me.' It's not as crazy as it seems, considering that just several weeks ago she had almost beaten me to death and that she had

undermined my relationship with my fiance. I cried out to my
father, 'Daddy, she's going to kill me!' "

New Diagnosis, More New Drugs

She agreed to go with her parents to the psychiatric ward at the
hospital. When she got there her mother told the psychiatrist that
she had delusions. She was diagnosed as a manic-depressive. She
refused to take the Lithium. They then changed her diagnosis to
'undifferentiated schizophrenia'. They tried to persuade her to
take Triliphon. She took one pill and she had to go to bed for two
days, she was so sick. She continued to refuse to take any drugs.
The doctors threatened to give her ECT but no action was taken.

While she was there a woman that she had become friendly
with committed suicide. This was right after the woman had
been given ECT. She'd jumped through a plate-glass window 15
minutes after the treatment and fell three stories to her death.
Kristin wanted to know what drug this woman had been on. She
asked the nurse if she could see the Physician's Desk Reference.
The nurse threatened to put her in seclusion.

They told her that if she did not take the Lithium she would
not be released from the hospital. So she took it.

> It made everything monotonous. I didn't care about anything.
> If someone had told me that my mother or father had died I
> would have just said, 'Hmm-mmm.' I couldn't get excited
> about anything. When I got out of the hospital they sent me to a
> mental health center. They said I'd have to take Lithium for the
> rest of my life. They said I was a manic-depressive.
> I said to them, "I've never been manic."
> They said, "Well, you're depressed, then."
> I said, "No, I'm not depressed, I'm sad."
> They can't understand that. It didn't meant that I was
> mentally ill or defective. It was natural for me to be sad. My
> marriage had failed, my parents sucked rocks, I had nowhere to
> go except back to the fiancé that I was fighting with because of
> my parents. What was I supposed to be so thrilled about?

The Expert: The denial of pathology demonstrates the fragili-
                ty of the patient's ego. She must accept that
                she must stay on Lithium for the rest of her

life in order to prevent a more serious decompensation. She will never be able to lead
a normal life or to have intimate heterosexual relationships. The damage is too severe
and the ego is not strong enough to withstand the re-activation of the initial transference. She should avoid over-stimulation and
be given supportive therapy to help her cope
and to form friendships that are not too de-
manding.

She moved in with one of her closest girlfriends. The woman
was divorced, with two kids. Kristin helped to take care of the
kids. "She made me feel it was nice to have me around. That was
the closest thing I'd had to having a family. I had never felt that
before. That was one of the happiest times of my life."

Kristin finished college and eventually moved several hours
away from her mother's home to go to graduate school. She
decided to get a master's degree in counseling. She thought that
she could work within the system to help people to change. She
finished her master's degree in two years and has been working as
a counselor for several years now. She has not taken any
psychiatric drugs since her last hospitalization, over eight years
ago.

She is not pleased with her job.

The mental health system has ripped me off twice, first as a
patient then as a counselor. I thought I could work within the
system. I was wrong. You can't show any human emotion
because they're mental-health trained. They look for symptoms
in everything and everybody, especially at work. They look
down on me because I was a mental patient. They even told me
not to tell any of the clients that I had ever been in a mental
hospital because the clients wouldn't respect me. Sometimes I
think I'm in a room filled with psychoanalysts and they're
analyzing me all day long. For example, they seem to have no
respect for the clients. All the things I feared that the mental
health professionals thought about us are worse than what I
thought it was from the other side. They think less of us and
more degrading of us than I would have ever imagined in my
most horrible dreams in the hospital. They've confirmed
everything I've ever dreaded.

One of the clients had gotten mad at one of the mental health workers because they were treating him in a condescending manner, as if he were a child. This 'patient', Conrad, said, "Just because I am a mental patient doesn't mean I don't know how to brush my teeth or shower, or that I can't take care of myself." So of course they said he had a paranoid delusion. The patient is paranoid if he or she thinks therapists talk about them. But we do. You do talk about them when they're gone. You all get together and talk about how paranoid they are that they think you're talking about them. It's crazy.

A psychiatrist said about this one patient who showed some independence, "He's a good paranoid schiz." I thought to myself, "Did you hear *anything* he said?" They didn't hear anything he said. And he quit today and I don't blame him. They engage continually in client-bashing in the treatment team. I brought in some writings that one of my clients had composed, and they just passed them around and they laughed and they laughed.

They listen to them in their sessions and they feel sorry for them but they basically don't care what they do with their lives. They don't help them to get their lives together.

Kristin feels that she has for the most part extricated herself from the marital triangle that her parents attempted to involve her in. She now lives three hours away from her parents and sees them less frequently. Sometimes she finds herself yearning once again for her parents' approval of what she's doing, but she is learning to break that habit and rely more on her own instincts. "If I tell my mother what I really feel about the mental health establishment she starts screaming, 'Wait a minute, wait a minute! You're supposed to be in the mental health establishment. You're just setting yourself up for a failure and you're going to end up back in the hospital and all this shit.' I can't talk to them at all."

She regrets that her parents do not have a more happy life together, but she knows that this is outside her power to change. Kristin is at a turning point in her life. From her own independent perspective, she sees all the flaws in the mental health system. She has developed the confidence to trust her own judgment and common sense.

She had escaped being inducted into the role of a chronic mental patient. But she is now stuck within a new role, a role with which she does not identify but which remains her source of livelihood. She is a social control agent whose job it is to attempt to induce individuals to accept the role of chronic mental patients. Her position in the agency is precarious and she refuses to perform this function and encourages 'patients' to become more independent. But she is keenly aware of the narrow limits of her power within a system that is organized in such a manner as to undermine individuals' confidence in their ability to function competently. Once again she is trapped and once again she is looking forward to the day when she will finally make her escape. She remains a rebel with a cause.

Six months after the above was written, Kristen left her job. "There was too much pressure on me to manipulate and intimidate the clients into taking drugs. When I helped people to get off drugs, the staff threatened to have me fired. I quit first."

Kristen has now been living with a new boyfriend for two years, and is happy in that relationship. She is about to commence a new career.

CHAPTER THREE

Cheryl's Story

I became acquainted with Cheryl after she heard me making a critique of the mental health system on the radio. After speaking with her briefly on the phone I sent her details of organized efforts to combat the system. I had mentioned that I was writing a book that consisted in part of former patients' stories. She wrote me a note thanking me for my response. She stated,

> Let me just say that I do have a horror story to tell but what I have that is more important is an analysis based not in anger or revenge but based on a respect for human rights. I truly feel a responsibility to the thousands of innocent victims of the psychiatric establishment. These people are voiceless and powerless against the machine that completely controls their lives in the name of 'help'. I want to do what I can to counteract this injustice and this violence.

Cheryl is an attractive, outgoing, affable, 36-year-old woman. She is happily married and the mother of an eight-year-old daughter. She is also a song-writer, a guitarist, and an activist in the movement for nuclear disarmament. She has been free of psychiatric drugs for 13 years. Like the many other individuals who fell into the net of the mental health establishment, she was told that she could not survive without Lithium.

Unhappy Childhood

Cheryl describes a troubled and miserable childhood. Her father had many breakdowns. She remembers vividly one incident that occurred when she was 16. This was the last time her father was home from the mental hospital before he died 10 years later in 1980.

> He took to his bed, would not get up, moaned, groaned, and was completely consumed by fear. He tried to cut his wrists in the presence of my sister and me.

44

The Expert: Both the genetic and the environmental variables create a strong predisposition towards
chronic schizophrenia, a debilitating disease
for which there is no cure. Psychiatric medication should be used to control the symptoms of the disease. The patient should not
be given false hopes and must realize that
she will never have a normal life.

Her father and her mother had rows whenever he was not
depressed. As Cheryl said, "It was either constant arguing or
depression." Despite the mental health experts' involvement in
her father's life, no attempt was made to protect Cheryl and her
two siblings. She lamented that there was a "lack of any kind of
cohesive family life".

Her older brother (by ten years) and her younger sister (by
three years) both tried to pretend that the problem did not exist.
Cheryl also tried this strategy at first. She withdrew to her room,
put a lock on her door, and tried to avoid her parents.

Dropping Out of College

In 1971 she entered City College. She was 17 and had always
been an excellent student. She continued to live at home and she
became increasingly depressed, to the point where she would not
function. The depression was severe and unrelenting.

> On my way to college, I would stand on the edge of the subway
> platform and literally want to jump off, to end my life. I
> thought about that 24 hours a day.

She would not continue college.

> I had to 'drop out' which was really, to a kid from Midwood
> High School in Brooklyn who always got A's, an honors
> student, one more nail in the coffin. A Jewish girl from
> Brooklyn, a good girl, a good student, and here she is quitting
> college. Oh, my God! Here I am depressed and this is some-
> thing to make me even more depressed.

She was frightened by what was happening to her. She felt as if
her brain had 'shut down'. She did not know what would happen
next.

> A person is functioning well and then all of a sudden they are overwhelmed by depression; they cannot move. I had seen my father turn into a vegetable over a long period of time. I was afraid this would happen to me.

Her mother was alarmed. Her mother conferred with Cheryl's brother, who had moved out of the house several years before, and with Cheryl's younger sister. They were all at a loss. They hoped she would 'snap out of it'.

Her father at this point had been put in a nursing home. She saw him as a victim of the mental health establishment. When she was young he worked at two jobs. He and her mother never talked.

> He came home at two or three in the morning, worked six days a week; the seventh day he watched baseball games with the transistor radio in one ear and the TV going on at the same time. So here was a man running from himself. He and my mother were completely estranged from one another. They stopped sleeping together from the time I was very small, so I never saw my mother and father together.

When he started to fall apart he became a pawn in the hands of the mental health establishment. The therapists made no attempt to foster communication between the couple, no attempt to bring out and negotiate the conflicts that had evidently led to her parents' emotional divorce from each other.

> My father was given every kind of drug. He was given every kind of diagnosis, several diagnoses. He was a schizophrenic, he was a psychotic, he was manic-depressive. There were so many doctors with so many different diagnoses and so many different medications. These people were playing Russian roulette. They had no idea what to do with the man so they labelled him and put him on drugs which eventually destroyed him.

The Expert: The patient's strong characterological defenses prevent her from accepting that her father suffered from a profound pathology. She utilizes the same mechanism of denial and blame in order to avoid acknowledging that she herself suffers from a chronic mental illness.

A Change of Mood

Her mother took her to an outpatient clinic where she was given 'medication'. No one talked to her or made any attempt to provide therapy. For several months she stayed depressed. Gradually the depression "started to pass".

> I became what they call 'manic'. And then I decided I was really going to live it up and I got myself a car. And I became extremely filled with my own power. I loved people. And I was very generous and I would run around and buy gifts for people and stay out late and meet new people. All of a sudden I was very popular. I started buying new clothes and looking good. What a contrast!

She did not know how to account for this change which happened rather suddenly.

She believed that her psyche was trying to compensate for her previous depression. It was as if her mind had spontaneously re-adjusted in order to permit her to enjoy life. She saw it as an adaptive response rather than as part of a pathological syndrome.

> Here I was wasting away and dying a slow death. And here some beautiful force was moving in to set me free. It was a gift.

The Expert: The patient utilizes denial and refuses to accept that she has a deeply rooted manic-depressive illness.

She was aware of both the negative and positive aspects of her new frame of mind.

> It was like a surge of life. It was a beautiful gift that felt very creative, very loving, but there was also a danger because your judgment is off. So I used to speed around in my car. I was a new driver.

Her family became very worried. This angered her because when she had been depressed no one had made serious efforts to find her any kind of help. "There was no great meeting or, 'Let's rush her into some program.' Their attitude was, 'She'll snap out of it.' And I felt abandoned."

The transformation in her personality aroused her family's greatest fears.

My brother was really worried about me. He said, "Give me a list of your friends and the phone numbers where I can reach you." Boy, was he nervous. Because, what a contrast! I was a quiet, nice, little girl who was depressed. They knew where I was because I was always sitting on the porch hunched over. They thought, 'We feel bad about it but at least we know where she is.'

Cheryl was describing one of the major impediments to the process of change: the fear of the unknown, the unanticipated, the unpredictable. Lacking the readiness to elicit 'unanticipated behavior', to "encourage unpredictability", as Jay Haley has put it, the professional becomes a social control agent whose goal is stability, rather than a therapist whose goal is transformation.

When Cheryl began to break out of her shell, the people around her became frightened.

It's frightening when somebody goes manic because they're unpredictable and not only that, they answer back. A depressed person accepts anything anyone says. If the doctor says, 'Take these pills', you take the pills. But a manic person is feisty.

She started working in her brother's business. When she was growing up she had been somewhat intimidated by her brother. Now she started to talk back to him and it was frightening to him. "It's upsetting to him. And he couldn't control it, he couldn't predict it."

I asked if she had been verbally abusive or violent.

No, I was not humiliating or cursing anyone out. I wasn't hitting anyone. I was being talkative, funny, popular, a little bit theatrical, dramatic . . . I was making up for all those years of being a mouse. All of a sudden, I was taking on parts of the personality I am today, 20 years later. In other words, my shyness had left me. But it was such an abrupt change, it was shocking and scary to people.

She felt that this was a liberating experience but she began to develop the sense that she was going too far and too fast.

A little voice was saying to me, 'This is not right. This is not really going to last. It's too fast, too soon, too much. You're spending all your money on presents for people.' A few people I knew were getting a little annoyed at me. Like, 'You're calling me at midnight to tell me you're coming over. I have to get up in the morning to go to work. Not everybody can get along without sleep.' In other words, a little voice started to tell me, 'This isn't right. You can't go on like this forever. You can't sustain this. You're starting to lose your friends. People are starting to shy away from you.' Because it's not natural. You can't cram a year's worth of life into a week.

The Expert: The patient is in the manic phase of her illness.

Tricked into the Mental Health System

At this point, fate intervened to bring events to a dramatic pitch. She was in a minor automobile accident that was not her fault. She went to her doctor who told her that she had a very slight concussion and that she should go home and rest. Her brother persuaded her to go to Mount Sinai Hospital for a second opinion. He led her into the hospital. She quickly discovered that he had tricked her and taken her to the psychiatric ward. She was committed against her will. She was told she was "one of the lucky ones" who was eligible for the experimental program with the new drug, Lithium. The psychiatrist told her that she was a manic-depressive like her father was. She was told that she was "genetically destined" to be ill for the rest of her life. She was told that this new drug would give her a chance to lead a normal life: it would control the symptoms of her disease.

I asked her how she felt about this.

> Part of me liked the fact that I was going to be helped and that since this was an experimental program, I would be used to help other people.

She became increasingly dissatisfied with the program. She fainted repeatedly from the Lithium. They had warned her of this possibility. Since Lithium is a highly toxic drug, they were constantly monitoring her blood levels. "My arms turned black and blue from all the tests they had to do." She did not like being confined. She felt humiliated by the way she was treated.

> In other words, I had to be controlled like a child. If I wanted to have my say, I was punished by extra sedatives. If I wanted to visit another patient and a staff member wanted me to go into my room and I didn't do what I was told, I would be threatened with more medication. Things like that. The nurses were treating us as if we were little, tiny children and they were omnipotent. And we had no rights; we had no human rights. We were constantly threatened with punishment, with isolation.

The Expert: The patient is unable to acknowledge, due to her
                 pathology, that her own lack of ego bound-
                 aries required that the staff impose limits on
                 her for her own protection.

She sneaked out of the hospital and took a cab to her friend
Lucy's house where she was a refugee for several weeks. Her
brother hired a detective to search for her. The detective came to
Lucy's house but Lucy refused to reveal any information. Cheryl
was afraid of being apprehended so she could not go out and find
work. Finally, she called her brother to tell him that she was safe.
Her brother instructed her to call her psychiatrist, Dr. Goldman,
at Mount Sinai. She called Dr. Goldman who told her that it was
essential that she came back for a blood test because the Lithium
was still in her system. Once again she was deceived and
committed against her will.
Cheryl believed they were vindictive about her escape.

> This time it was hardball; this time it was heavy Thorazine.
> Heavy. My eyesight went. I could not read even large print. It
> was terrifying. My hands shook, I couldn't even pour a glass of
> juice. I could not hold anything hot because I would probably
> scald myself. It was as if I was slowly but surely losing my
> ability to function as a human being. My brother, the man who
> had put me away to begin with, became horrified. He signed me
> out of the hospital against Dr. Goldman's orders.

I asked her what frightened her brother.

> I could not recognize my own brother. My muscles were
> twitching from the drugs. Later my brother told me that he said
> to a private psychiatrist he consulted, "I was scared when I saw
> my sister. She didn't know me." The psychiatrist told him they
> were a bunch of crazies over there.

Her brother arranged for Cheryl to have sessions with a
psychiatrist whom he knew. He placed her in an apartment with
a room-mate who was a patient of this psychiatrist. "I became
more and more angry at my brother, with the way he was trying
to control me. Also, he was paying my room-mate to keep an eye
on me."
She refused to continue going to see the psychiatrist. She told
her brother to "go to hell" and he was enraged. Once again he
asked her if she would take a little drive with him. He wanted her
just to have a talk with a different therapist. He took her to

King's County Hospital where she was committed against her will. She was furious at herself for trusting her brother again.

She made an effort to persuade the psychiatrist that she was not insane and ought not to be committed.

> I spoke with intense deliberation trying to convince him of my sanity. I said "Doctor, I am absolutely in control of my mind." There was a blank expression on his face. I found out later that my psychiatrist had already talked to him. If your sanity is being questioned, then there is nothing you can do to prove you're sane. You can't talk your way out of it. I pleaded with him. I begged him. Then I realized that I was there to be committed. My destiny was planned. There was nothing I could do in that space of time to change the verdict.

A woman came in with a set of keys and started to lead her away. She followed reluctantly. She was taken to a ward where there were many people classified as criminally insane. She was to be held there temporarily until they found the appropriate ward for her. She was given an injection of drugs. She felt dazed. She looked around the room and she was horrified. It was a huge room. There were two large guards with guns. People were howling and screaming. Many were in straitjackets. "I could not believe that this was happening in New York. It was as if I walked into Hell, Hell on Earth."

After a day she called her mother and told her that she intended to jump out the window if her mother did not come down there immediately. Her mother came down and facilitated her immediate transfer to another ward. Once she was on this ward, she decided to be as obedient as possible in order to be released as quickly as possible. The medication made her feel "foggy", "dull", and "sluggish". It was difficult to move and to co-ordinate her movements. She saw many patients who refused to take the pills. They were forcibly injected. Cheryl 'behaved'. "I served my sentence." Three weeks later she was released.

After she was released from the hospital she went to her family physician who said to her, "Cheryl, you are toxic. Get off these drugs. Get some rest and eat well." She stayed with her mother for a while. She was having trouble getting her energy back. She had discontinued seeing a psychiatrist or taking psychiatric drugs.

She expressed her criticisms of her treatment.

> I went into the mental health system and I did not get any therapy, any guidance. No one gave me any insight into how

growing up in a dysfunctional family for 18 years would have an impact on my present life. I had been in two different hospitals. I had spoken to countless psychiatrists and not once did I find someone who gave me any insight. Not once did I find anyone who treated me as if I was on his level. No, I was mentally sick and they were well. I was told over and over again that I had a disease like diabetes. I wasn't given a chance. They did not even open up one door for me. The crime was not just all the harmful, frightening things they did to me, like taking away my freedom and giving me drugs that turned me into a zombie. The crime was also what they failed to do, the genuine help that they might have provided, but did not provide.

Despite recurrent periods of depression between 1972 and 1978, she stayed away from the mental health system and off of psychiatric drugs. She worked full-time as a typesetter. In 1972 she met the man whom she would marry two years later. Despite the past, she felt strongly bonded to her husband. They had marital conflicts which led to a separation in 1978. She was troubled by feelings of loneliness and despair. She felt she was just surviving. "I'm a Leo. I'm not meant to be just a surviving person. I'm meant to be dynamic, to have drama in my life."

Attempt at Suicide

She thought of consulting a therapist but was worried because of her negative experiences in the past. Finally, in 1978, she went to a psychiatrist who suggested she go on antidepressant 'medication'. She complied. Once again her feelings of discouragement were attributed to an ostensibly defective genetic system. Although this psychiatrist encouraged her to talk about the past, she knew that he viewed her as a defective person. His lack of confidence in her made her leery. It did not occur to him that Cheryl's feelings of despair may have been a natural response to events in her life—her current estrangement from her husband, as well as traumas suffered as a child. She discontinued therapy.

She was lonely and apathetic. In 1980 her father died. He passed away in a mental hospital. She visited him shortly before he died. "I saw him turn white." She moved to Florida to live with an aunt. She missed her husband. She was devastated by her father's death. "I gave up hope. I thought, 'I cannot take this anymore.'" She had reached the 'bottom' of her life. She was determined to die. The intensity of the depression was worse than anything she had ever experienced before. "I went to a hotel room in a strange city, closed the door, and took a bottle of pills, enough pills to kill me." Somehow she was discovered.

She woke up in a hospital. She was no longer depressed. She was happy to be alive. "I feel a miracle happened to me, a miracle. I was shocked. I felt different. I was completely lifted out of doom."

"By God?" I asked.

"Of course. I was meant to be alive. And I took that as a sign that nothing was going to be the same again and nothing was. I'm living under grace now."

The Expert: Religious delusions are a typical sign of a psychotic disorder. The ideas of reference and the feelings of grandiosity the patient expresses are a reaction formation to the low sense of self-worth she experiences as a result of severe ego defects.

When she was released from the hospital, she went back to live with her aunt. They had persuaded her to participate in outpatient care and to take Lithium. "I was scared and so I complied. They told me that I would try to commit suicide again if I went off the Lithium. Along with the Lithium, they give you a big dose of fear. They acted as if they were God."

She went for regular blood tests and participated in the out-patient group for manic-depressives. "It's so superficial. All you talk about is the medication. You don't talk about your life. The therapist says, 'Is the medication working? See you next time.'"

Breaking Free

Meanwhile she had been talking to her husband who wanted to try to work things out with her. He wanted her to move back to New York and live with him. He also wanted her to stop taking Lithium. "He had an intuitive sense that it was dangerous, a false promise. He said it does not belong in your body. He had confidence in me—that I could handle life without Lithium. He gave me inspiration and courage."

Cheryl decided that she was going to go to the heads of the

out-patient program and tell them that she was going off of Lithium, that she was quitting the program, and that she was going back to New York to live with her husband.

> They went hysterical. "You cannot do this," they said. "You'll be depressed. You'll try to commit suicide. We're warning you," they said. "You'll regret it." Well, I have never regretted it. I'm only thankful that my husband was the one person in my life to have faith in me. It's been ten years since I've been off Lithium and I have not regretted it once. In fact, I have not been seriously depressed since then. Having the baby had a lot to do with it. It gave me a new love in my life, a new source of life.

She moved back in with her husband and one month later she became pregnant. If she had stayed on Lithium, she would have had to have an abortion. She also began to study the guitar, make new friends, and become an activist in the nuclear disarmament movement.

Although 1980 through 1987 was basically a happy period for Cheryl, she continued to be troubled from time to time by the ghosts in her past. She felt that her union with her husband was impeded by fears and phantasies that stemmed from her childhood and adolescence. She learned this when she went into therapy in 1987 with a woman she felt she could trust. This had a positive effect on her relationship with her husband.

> When I have a problem with my husband, consciously I'm mad at my husband but unconsciously I may be mad at my father. You see then I can become aware of feeling abandoned by my father. And I do a meditation and I visualize my father and I forgive him and these feelings disappear. It's amazing. I'm healing something. And I wake up the next day and all the negative feelings are gone.

This happens frequently: she realizes that she is feeling resentful at her husband and he has done nothing wrong.

> And I say, "Wait a minute, Cheryl. Don't let this *run you*." And I do a meditation. There are certain skills you can develop. You don't have to take a pill. You don't have to check into a hospital.

Whereas before she was controlled by the thoughts and fears that were triggered in her mind by various stimuli, now she can monitor and control her thoughts so that she does not become overwhelmed by feelings of despair. "I learned through therapy that I do not have to accept every negative thought that comes into my head. There are ways to change your thoughts and calm yourself down."

Among the negative thoughts that used to 'run' her were the ones that the mental health establishment attempted to inculcate in her: that she was genetically damaged, that she was inferior, that she had a 'disease' like diabetes.

> You know, that was their frame-up. They branded me. I started to think, 'I really am mentally sick.' They do that to you and people believe what they say because they are doctors. My therapist helped make me aware that I am not damaged goods, that I really am whole, worthy of love, even when I am having a problem.

She was in therapy from 1987 to 1989. She believes that her therapist helped her to accept and forgive her mother and father for their failure to provide her with the support she would have liked as a child. Cheryl started therapy shortly after her mother had a heart attack in 1987. "I realized the need to forgive my mother and father to break free of anger and guilt."

Her mother died in 1988. She believes that her brother and sister, both of whom are apparently successful and without any history of breakdowns, have never resolved their feelings of abandonment and anger towards their parents. Cheryl said,

> When my mother died, I sent my sister a photograph and some artifacts of my mother. She put them in a drawer. Nothing in her apartment even indicates that she had a mother. I love my mother. I'm proud of her. I know she had a hard time and she could be said to have failed us in many ways, but she did the best she knew how. And she was a great woman, an entertainer.

She believes that her brother and sister are still refusing to acknowledge their pain. Her sister now has some unexplained depression. "She never had the crisis I had. So in a way, I'm more thankful because I was able to go through the pain and find some answers."

On the other hand she avoided the fate of many of her peers in mental hospitals:

> I saw beautiful young people put away in state mental hospitals. I saw many young girls crying when they heard they were being sent to a state institution. I'm grateful: I had the groundwork laid where I could be following in the footsteps of those professional mental patients. Instead I'm a mother, a social activist, a songwriter. I'm not on drugs. I'm a survivor. I'm happy. I'm not manic. I'm thankful to be alive.

CHAPTER FOUR

Ruby's Story

I met Ruby at a party. She is a tall, light-skinned black woman. We went out and talked informally several times. A year later she agreed to be interviewed by me. She felt that she had proven the Mental Health Establishment wrong.

The story begins when she was about to leave high school. She had been in a lesbian relationship for six years, from age 16 to 22. She wanted to end the relationship and divorce herself from the lesbian subculture she had drifted into. "I felt that it wasn't really who I wanted to be." She had strong romantic and sexual phantasies about men and she wanted to make the transition to a heterosexual lifestyle. However there was no one to support her in making the transition.

The Expert: The patient is an ego-dystonic homosexual. This is a serious disorder that can be alleviated somewhat with the help of supportive therapy. Her ego defects prevent her from accepting her homosexuality.

She felt that there was no one she could talk to about her dilemma:

> I couldn't talk to my gay and lesbian friends because they would have been mortified if I said I wanted to date men. All they kept doing was pushing me back into a gay and lesbian mentality. I said I was attracted to men. They said, 'That's only because you've been raised in a straight society. And that's only because you've been conditioned to want men.' They kept trivializing everything I was saying. I said, 'I'm telling you. I always phantasize about men.' 'But that's only because you're trying to have a straight identity.' And they would almost convince me. But I'd think, 'That's just not it.' And so there were none of my friends that I could talk to about it, because I knew that they would chastise me, they wouldn't speak to me again. It was a threat to the gay and lesbian community, especially at this time because of AIDS.

56

Uncertain Orientation

Her feelings were ambivalent. Although she was romantically drawn to men, she could think of many reasons why she ought to avoid becoming sexually involved with a man:

> Logically it didn't make sense to me to want men. Men make more money. They have more power and they're abusive because they have more power. I had been abused by them. They're physically stronger; they can beat me up. Why should anyone want that? But as time goes on, desire has become very complex; it's not that easy. Why do we want one person? It's very complicated.

Her anguish was intensified by the fact that there was no one she could talk to. "You know it would have made a big difference if I could have developed trust with someone enough to feel that I could have talked to him or her." She believed that if she had gone to a therapist, the therapist would have treated her as if she were a homosexual who would not accept her homosexuality.

> They would have labelled me an ego-dystonic homosexual. They pretend to be hip now, so they say it's normal to be homosexual. Of course, they don't think it's normal at all, but that's what they're giving lip service to these days. But they think you're even more abnormal if you do not accept your abnormality.

Part of the problem was that the transition she wanted to make was unusual.

> People don't go from gay to straight. It's so hard to explain, but there was just no way to say it without being pushed back into, 'You're really gay and just won't accept it.' It would have been like pushing up against a wall.

She felt that she was living a lie.

> My whole lifestyle was giving a lot of lip service to lesbian rights, and I was one hundred percent behind the community. They would say 'Gay Rights' and I'd raise my fist in approval and say 'Right on!' But in my mind I wanted to go out with the guy sitting next to me.

She described a particularly intense experience she had with a man she had been friends with for a long time. He was one of her best friends. Her phantasies in the past had been mostly about male rock stars—not really particularly accessible. But on this occasion, fantasy and reality melded together. She was sitting with her friend.

> All of a sudden I made the connection. It was almost as if I had an image of Cupid shooting an arrow into my heart. The room lit up; I saw him through rose-colored lenses. It's hard to describe. Forgive the clichés but I felt like, 'Wow!' It blew my mind. It was just like the movies. I thought 'I'm falling in love.' He looked at me and I looked at him and I thought, 'This is real. Don't just phantasize about these things. Go after the one you're phantasizing about.' It's not authentic to have such strong romantic feelings for men and to be going out with women. The hell with being politically correct.

I asked her if she consummated the relationship with her friend.

> No, I couldn't. I couldn't deal with it at all. This was when I started to become psychotic. I was bombarded with thoughts like, 'Do I want to find a man now?' And I always felt I would. 'But can I have a relationship? Is he going to hit me?' I mean when I say that, my mind started going around and around at 100 miles an hour. I had never had a boyfriend, really. I mean I had had a few boyfriends when I was younger but I never had an ongoing sexual relationship. So I had performance anxiety. I thought, 'I won't be good in bed with a man.' I'd slept with a lot of men but I'd never had an ongoing relationship where you learned how to make love. I was bombarded with every single nutty thought that you could ever have, in one fell swoop: 'He's gonna beat me. I can't do this. He's gonna hurt me. I can't sleep with him. What if he's the one I want? Does that mean I have to get married? I don't want to have children. Can my friends accept this? How will I get out of my relationship with Ann. And how am I gonna . . .'—and on and on. My mind went around and around. I couldn't turn it off.

Evidently, the more real the possibility became of having a relationship with a man, the more the fears and potential obstacles came to the surface. It is instructive to remember here that moving ahead to a new phase of the life cycle can precipitate a developmental crisis, as Jay Haley has pointed out repeatedly. The void of the unknown becomes filled with ghosts and phantasies from the past.

Crisis and Hospitalization

Growing up at home had been intensely nerve-racking for Ruby. The real issues between her parents were never debated openly. Eventually, they stopped sleeping together.

> My father was utterly explosive. You were always walking on eggshells. My parents were always on the verge of splitting up. What kept them together, I think, was the sense that they were allies in a world that was against them. But the love had gone.

She decided to leave the gay subculture, but she was frightened of the challenge of dealing with men. Her lover, Ann, clung to her and did not want to terminate the relationship. A friend of Ruby's had died in the streets and Ruby felt that her friend might not have died had Ruby been more responsive to her.

> I was between a rock and a hard place. I was trapped in a lifestyle that I definitely wanted out of and I couldn't see any way to wipe it out. So in some way I felt that going mad was my choice, because it almost seemed to wipe out everything. I could remember at times almost *acting* crazy. I told that to my shrink and he thought that was stupid.

In the beginning it felt as if she had no control. Everything just fell apart.

> It was madness, it was wild. I was hearing voices. I had met this guy I was attracted to and I started thinking he was trying to kill me. He was my sister's room-mate. She threw him out because she believed me. I became increasingly more paranoid. I'd go to work and I'd think people were staring at me and talking about me. I was 23 at the time. I was still able to work and function. I started working as a receptionist in a law firm. And I got a crush on one of the lawyers there and eventually, I would hear his voice all the time. I could function with the voices but I started thinking, 'Maybe I'm really dangerous.' In August 1984, I decided to sign myself into Bellevue.

She was in the hospital for a month. She did not tell anyone about her homosexual relationship because she believed they would then say, 'Clearly, she's a lesbian. And that is why she's having all these problems.'

> And I didn't want that. I felt they would invalidate what I was fantasizing about and wanted to be. And I felt I should have the right to choose my own lifestyle.

After being in the hospital for two weeks, she decided she wanted to leave. She had signed herself in voluntarily. At this point two psychiatrists examined her, declared that she was a danger to herself and others, and consequently could not leave the hospital. Up until this point she had felt relatively safe in the hospital. Now she started to feel rebellious. And yet at the same time she wanted help.

Ruby felt that the experience of madness made her aware of another dimension of human existence, one which the psychiatrists and normal people seem oblivious to.

> The one thing that happened to me by becoming crazy, and why I will never be 'normal' by other people's standards, is that that experience is very much like near-death experiences. We cannot go back to being as we were before, because it's the kind of experience that brings you to a different consciousness. When what Garfinkle calls the 'taken-for-granted reality' gets all shaken up, it's never the same. You can't just go back to picking daisies in the park.

She saw that reality was something that could be taken apart and 'remade'.

> My whole reality was something that I constructed and had nothing to do with what I felt. I had constructed a whole reality with words, with nothing but words, that were utterly meaningless. They had no relationship to what I was feeling at all. And the whole world that I had created just fell apart.

Her self-identity as a lesbian was experienced as a facade. She had played a part and then she became the character she was playing. Now she was plunged into chaos. Who was she? What was she experiencing? Eliade has written of the return to primordial chaos that precedes a new creation, a creation more consonant with the deeper, more authentic yearnings of the self. But there was no one there to guide her. She had not yet read R.D. Laing, who had written: "Madness need not be all breakdown. It may also be breakthrough. It is potentially liberation and renewal as well as enslavement and existential death."

> There was nobody there giving me any framework to put this in. I had nothing to make sense out of it on any level. So it really was just chaos. I was going round in circles. It was madness. It was wild.

Breakthrough

On the one hand, chaos, and on the other hand, the awareness that the mind can give substance to a reality, to a fictive reality. She was frightened by the power of the mind.

> I have become so truthful because I am afraid of the fact that if I just tell a lie, I can totally shift the reality. If I go into a room where no one knows me and I tell these people I'm an actress, they'll believe me and they'll act on that. And in that room, I can create a whole other reality.

But is everything totally fictive, an arbitrary creation *ex nihilo?* Was everything ultimately illusory? She emerged from the experience with the sense that there was an authentic dimension to the self: words and images that reflected the self without distortion. But in the midst of her breakdown she was aware of the threat of nothingness. "I felt as if I was going to unravel to the point where there was no I, me, or anything; there was just no consciousness at all. So what I held onto were the eternal truths."

The Expert: The patient has decompensated totally as a result of homosexual panic. The fragility of her ego boundaries, the regression to a primitive pre-verbal mode of experience, the recurrent feelings of infantile omnipotence are clearly symptoms of a deep pathology. The character disorder manifested in her inability to accept her homosexuality is secondary to the evident diagnosis of chronic schizophrenia. The patient should be maintained on anti-psychotic medication and learn to accept that she will never be able to lead a normal life. Supportive therapy should be provided to help her accept her homosexuality. Her repeated failure to make a satisfactory heterosexual adjustment must be gently pointed out to her.

I asked her what were the eternal truths:

> I live. I die. I was very in touch with my own mortality. And in that sense, I felt what you called a sense of oneness with the

human race. What have people grappled with since the beginning of time? Our mortality, trying to somehow get beyond our mortality.

"Do you mean," I asked, "a sense that humanity is united under the curse of death?"

Yes, that's exactly right. That was how I saw us as one. I went to look at the tombs in Egypt. 'My God,' I thought, 'this is a desperate attempt to gain control of death, just struggling to gain control over something that ultimately we don't have the control over.'

"I believe it is ultimately our destiny as a species to transcend physical mortality. That this is not a law of nature but a manifestation of our estrangement from God," I told her.

When she was reflecting on these issues in the hospital, she began to realize that her psychiatrists were themselves out of touch with reality. If one faces fully the horror of death, is it not natural to go mad? "I think that to fully understand our mortality is to be mad. To come to grips with our mortality is just maddening, isn't it?"

I replied: "Those who are more aware of death may go crazy and then get labelled mentally ill by the psychiatrists whose strategy is to pretend that death doesn't exist."

Psychiatry thinks that fear of death is a symptom of a mental illness! You start thinking, 'Okay, who is crazy here?' You start realizing the craziness of everyone around you. And I think I needed to see that because it broke down the us-and-them barrier. I thought, 'We are the ones who are crazy and they're normal? Let's face it we're all out of our fucking minds here. We're bananas.'

The time in the hospital was "not so bad" because all the time she was thinking, 'Maybe this will allow me to make the transition. It was only four or five weeks. And I felt like maybe this is what I needed.' She did however object to the strong doses of psychiatric drugs which slowed her down and made her feel straitjacketed.

When she left she was "hopeful". She went to school to register. Her hands were shaking and she felt anxious. She went to live with her parents. And then she went to see a psychiatrist, "this horrible quack", Dr. Crouther.

She was rigid; she was cold. And she hated me for not being rigid and cold. She just sat there without responding. At the

> second meeting she declared, "Well I've heard what you've had to say, and I've read your file. And I've diagnosed you as a paranoid-schizophrenic." I absolutely flipped. It invalidated me. I was not a person. She had just told me point blank, 'You are not a person. You were born defective and that's it. You would have lived a crazy life no matter what had happened to you, you would have ended up at the same point, because you are defective.'

Instead of helping the person to resolve their life crises, the therapist becomes another problem to contend with. The therapist seeks to undermine the person's self-respect. The life issues that a person is grappling with are obscured.

> She never once asked me about my life. She never once asked me what I was feeling. She just wanted to know, 'Are you taking your drugs?' and absolutely tuned out if I talked about anything else. She just didn't believe in me. She couldn't see me. All she saw was a label. I brought my mother in. My mother said, 'You don't know anything about her. She was the smartest kid in school. She went to Bronx Science which is a very competitive school.'

The Expert: The fragility of the patient's ego is evidenced by her inability to accept her pathology. Her feelings of hostility are disowned and projected onto her therapist who is construed as an aggressive 'bad mother'.

Even when her psychiatrist did not talk, Ruby sensed that she regarded her as sick.

> I used to go in there and try to argue with her and she just dismissed everything I said. She never responded, as if everything I said was just more evidence of my pathology. She just kind of stared at me, like, 'Um-hmm.' As if my words had no meaning.

The psychiatrist tried to discourage her from returning to school. She said, "I think you really shouldn't. You won't be able to handle it and you should really take it easy."

Ruby might have been inducted into the role of a professional mental patient but she had too much self-respect. She was too independent a spirit to conform to the mental health establishment's limited view of who she was and who she would become.

I went to school and I just pushed myself. I was determined to prove it to myself and to them. I wanted to show that I could be normal like everyone else, 'There's so much more to who I am than what you allow yourself to see.' I wanted to say to the psychiatrists, 'Stop saying "You poor victim" and that condescending garbage.' They try to act like they're on your side and that you're crazy because you won't accept their kindness. I feel like, 'You've got to be kidding. This is the most condescending thing I've ever heard in my life.'

She knew a lot of people who became professional mental patients, who "totally buy into" being mentally ill.

They don't want to do anything. They get money from the government, they get pity wherever they go, and they get lots of attention from the professionals. People talk to them who ordinarily would never walk down the same side of the street with them. I don't fault them because no one is helping them develop a critical consciousness at all. But I was willing to say, "Shove this. I don't accept that I'm a hopeless schizophrenic" and to start looking around for alternative viewpoints. You know, I read this article, "Mental Patients Who Don't Like Psychiatrists" and it said they don't have a strong identity and they split, etc. etc. So I did a little survey on my own and I found that overwhelmingly, SSI was a deciding factor. If you got no SSI, you hated psychiatry. If you got SSI, you liked psychiatry. There are benefits to buying into the system."

Ruby is now completing her master's in social work. She intends to be a community organizer. She studies hard. "I wanted to prove to myself and to the people around me that I can do this. 'Don't condescend to me and act like you're doing me a favor.'"

She sees the positive side of going mad: it allowed her to break out of a mould that was constraining her and to create a new identity for herself. She has a number of friends now and she occasionally dates men but she has not yet been involved in an ongoing intimate relationship. She still phantasizes about being with a man, but feels insecure on that score.

"That's common," I said.

"Well, having been in a mental hospital does not help."

She still takes a low dosage of a neuroleptic drug. She takes, in fact, half the amount that the manufacturer states is necessary to be effective.

I said that many people find neuroleptics impede their creativity.

"Yes, on higher dosages that is true. But on low dosages, it helps you to sleep."

Recapitulation

What happened? She went mad. But did she go mad because she has a disease called schizophrenia? She went mad because she was faced with extraordinary challenges because she was contemplating making a major change in her mode of being.

Ultimately, what was at stake was her sense of personal identity: "I felt as if I was going to unravel to the point where there was no I." One might speculate: the sense of a future, rife with new possibilities caused and demanded this divesture of self. Eliade writes, "The initiatory death repeats this exemplary return to Chaos in order to make possible a renewal of the cosmogony; that is, to prepare for the new birth."[1] He notes that this often involves a total "disintegration of the personality".

While later Ruby would speak of living a "lie", in the midst of her madness, any expression of the self must have seemed to be fictive: homosexuality, heterosexuality, bisexuality. The distinction between truth and falsehood is obliterated in the moment of crisis of madness. As she put it: it is "wild". There is nothing that authorizes the productions of the person. Later she rediscovered a consonance between her words and actions and her being. In Jungian terms, one might say that the ego, the outer personality, was repossessed by the Self, the invisible author that grants the gift of form and meaning to the conscious mind (the ego) strong enough to receive its images and inspirations. Retrospectively Ruby perceives the dissonance that had existed between her words and her inner yearnings. "I had constructed a whole reality with words . . . They had no relationship to what I was feeling at all." She has now achieved a poise that feels authentic.

In the moment of madness, she became aware of the reality of physical mortality and she was shocked by the smugness of the mental health professionals. "Psychiatry thinks that fear of death is a syndrome." Like R.D. Laing, she realizes that her doctors were in a state of oblivion far more dangerous than the madness that may possess a person who strives to remain true to herself.

[1]Mircea Eliade, *Myths, Dreams, and Mysteries* (New York: Harper and Row, 1975), 224

Barbara's Story

Barbara is a 35-year-old woman who grew up in Texas and lives there today. I became acquainted with her by telephone after she had seen me on TV and called to inquire about our organization. She is the mother of a 15-year-old son, the survivor of three psychiatric incarcerations, and an activist in the movement against psychiatric oppression.

This is the story of a young woman growing up in a less than ideal world, contending with the various challenges of life and emerging triumphant, with a sense of self-respect that has grown stronger despite the various assaults on her being.

The mental health establishment attributes all of a person's struggles to a putative defective internal system. External factors that could account for the person's unease are ignored. The premise is: there is something wrong with you. All of the data are then organized in such a way that it seems to validate that premise. The experts *selectively* focus on individuals' 'failures', interpret them as symptoms of illnesses and then inform them that they are permanently doomed to lead a marginal existence. Millions of individuals succumb to the spell of this curse. Barbara did not.

Unfulfilling Childhood

What follows is not the story of a defective woman but of a woman relentlessly struggling to overcome the obstacles to the realization of her aspirations. "Life is not a walk across an open field," Pasternak writes. If it were an open field one might cogently construe the difficulties Barbara experienced as evidence that she suffered from some internal mental defect. As it is, this construction was merely another obstacle placed in her path by experts who attempted to undermine her self-confidence in the name of protecting her mental health.

Barbara's childhood was lonely and unfulfilling. Her mother and her father did not get along well. He was domineering, and physically abusive on several occasions. This stopped after Barbara's mother, Mary, bought a gun and told him she would kill him if he ever touched her again. There was little communication between the two of them.

Mary had a closer relationship with Barbara than she did with her husband. "She trusted me. She did not trust him." Barbara was the only one who knew about Mary's affairs. Barbara's brother was six years older and stayed aloof from the family.

Barbara finished high school and married a man in the army when she was 17. Two years later her son Gerald was born. The marriage was "Hell". "He wanted a live-in housekeeper. There was no emotional sharing. He would get angry at me if I tried to get a conversation going about anything more than superficial." She got a divorce.

The next several years were barren and lonely. Her energy went into caring for and raising her son. She lived in a house behind her mother's who would call her every night to see if she was home safe. "I didn't date, I didn't do anything but raise my son."

The Expert: The patient suffers from a borderline personality disorder. Her inability to form social relationships is evidence of the fragility of her self-concept. The characterological defect is manifested by the denial of her pathology. Oral deprivation at an early age has created excessive dependency needs that prevent her from being fulfilled by her husband. Due to the intensity of her transference her husband is experienced as a withholding mother.

Gradually she began to distance herself from her mother. She took very seriously her own responsibilities as a mother and she became skeptical of her mother's advice. "When my son began to show signs of getting sick physically I recognized that she was causing it and I started telling her to leave him alone."

If Gerald sneezed, Mary would say, 'I think he's got a fever. I think he's getting sick.' And then Barbara would worry. "And then he would just comply and get real sick." She started to realize that she knew better than her mother.

She got a job at a custom photography studio where she worked for a couple of years. She quit because she was disturbed by the fact that her boss who was married was carrying on a clandestine affair with his secretary.

A New Relationship

She was exercising regularly and losing weight when she started to look for another job, which she found at a newspaper office. She was 27. It was there that she met Daniel, with whom she fell in love. She moved in with him. "He was a person who considered himself a wizard and a mystic." In the beginning of the relationship she would try to please and appease him all the time.

They started their own local newspaper together which became very successful. She was the editor, she developed the photographs, she wrote a column every week. "It gave me the realization that I was competent in a workaday world."

Tensions in the relationship increased. "Sex was constantly on his mind." He wanted Barbara to act out the fantasy he had of seeing two lesbians make love to each other. First he pressured her to read stories out of the porno magazines he had. Then he wanted her to make stories up. "I felt very used. He said he would leave me if I did not comply. The tension was so high in me that I wanted to scream all the time."

The Expert: Low tolerance for frustration is typical of the
                 borderline personality disorder. Her failure
                 to terminate the relationship is symptomatic
                 of excessive dependency needs.

I asked Barbara why she wanted to maintain the relationship. She responded, "He was very intelligent and interesting. He was more affectionate than any man I'd ever been with, without sex even. He'd hold my hand and he'd put his arm around me while we were out in public, as if to say, 'This woman is my woman', and that made me feel I belonged with him." She had met Daniel when she was 27 and now she was 29.

During these years she had disengaged herself from her relationship with her mother and they were now on better terms. Barbara was working full-time and she had demonstrated that she was a sensitive and competent mother. She had more self-confidence than ever before. "I began to stand up to him and say, "I'm not going to do these things that I don't like to do.

You're not God; you're not so smart as you think you are.' I fully thought we could have an open conversation and put the facts out on the table and work them out. Because we were married and I thought that he was going to stick with me no matter what."

Daniel became increasingly disturbed by Barbara's independence. "What frightened him was that I was not compliant any more, that I could resist, that I could protest. And he had lost control of me. And if he could not control me I suppose he was afraid he would be controlled."

"Or abandoned," I suggested.

"Yes, or abandoned. Because one time I got angry and went for a walk and he comes running out there looking for me and he says, 'Please don't ever leave me.' But after that it was like he was on his way out."

I responded, "The idea is, 'If I leave her before she leaves me I feel safer.'"

"Yes, that was exactly it. Because he just left, abandoned me and my son who regarded him as his father. He'd call me up occasionally and say he might come back but he wouldn't say where he was. That was one of the worst experiences I have ever been through in my life."

The Expert: The transferential feelings towards her husband and her weak ego boundaries lead her to regress to the early stage of infancy. The patient is not capable of handling the demands of adult life due to the severity of her pathology. She should be given medication and supportive therapy and be helped to avoid interpersonal relationships that might activate the transference and lead to the threat of decompensation.

Visions and Messages

Barbara had no one to tell her troubles to. She felt miserably alone. She had been taking a small amount of Ativan for over a year now, to help decrease the anxiety she felt as a result of tensions in her life. She stopped taking all drugs. "I got more and more to where I just could not sleep at night. I was constantly on edge, waiting, looking, hoping I'd see his vehicle coming up the road."

And one night I was outside sweeping off the deck and something made me look up, and I saw this light that appeared to be rising in the sky. And I thought it was an airplane, and when it stopped moving I thought still that it was an airplane and it had just leveled off. But the thing didn't move any more, it just sat there. And I started feeling what I call 'the tinglies' from the top of my head to the bottom of my feet, just flowing back and forth through me. And I felt very, very happy. And I felt like whoever—I felt like there was a 'who' rather than a 'what'—was at that light was aware of me.

"Do you think that was an extraterrestrial or something?," I asked?

Well, at the time I thought it was a star. I wasn't into UFOs yet. But now I do believe it was extraterrestrial. It just stayed up there in the sky for at least a half an hour before I stopped looking at it. And I had my son come out, because I had begun to be afraid I was gonna go nuts, and I didn't want to be hallucinating. So I asked him what he saw up there and he described what he saw, so I knew he saw what I saw. He also pointed out later that he had noted there were two other lights below that, to the left and the right, so that they would form a triangle. I hadn't seen those.

"So what possible explanation is there, other than that it was some kind of extraterrestrial object?" I asked.

Nothing, because there was no sound, and it was too big. It was very large in comparison to the stars, which meant it was closer. And I don't know of any planes or any kind of aircraft that we have that can just sit there quietly with a light. And weather balloons don't do that. And I know I've seen a couple of lights since then, and Wimberly is a pretty good place for it. There are a lot of people who have reported UFO sightings around here. That gave me a sense of wonder and happiness. It didn't last, because there was still the problem with 'Where's my husband? Where's my husband?'

She was till barely able to sleep. She began to have 'visions'. "I was aware of synchronistic events occurring rapidly, one right after the other, constantly. Television, the radio, books, anything was a sign of something other than its surface value. And it was very exciting to me."

The Expert: The patient has lost touch with reality and is in the beginning phase of a schizophrenic episode.

I responded, "Jung's idea of synchronicity posits a universe that is continually giving messages to us—if only we'd listen."

"That's what Carlos Castañeda says also. Because Don Juan, the shaman, the spiritual teacher, would be talking to Carlos and an airplane would fly over and he'd say, 'See, the world agrees with me.' "

I asked her to give an example from her experience. "I went to turn the television off and something, I got a message to turn the television back on."

"How was the message conveyed?" I asked.

> It was like a thought in my mind. I turned it back on and there was a commercial—or something, I can't exactly remember—but whatever it was I got the impression to go outside and raise the hood of my truck. Because this morning I had tried to go somewhere and the truck wouldn't start. That was in the morning and now it was in the middle of the afternoon. Now I thought to myself, 'Why? What purpose?' Because I don't know how to fix a truck. But I knew, 'Okay, that's what I'm supposed to do.' So I walked outside and I raised the hood of my truck and I went back in the house and within two minutes I heard a truck coming down the road and it was my neighbor, coming home in the middle of the day, which he never did. And he comes rattling up the road and he sees the hood of my truck open so he pulls into my driveway. And he jumpstarts my truck. He gets it running so I could go into town. And I understood what the whole thing was about.

"As if one listens to the messages of the universe one would get assistance and things would work out effortlessly?"

"Yes, but of course I didn't think of it in those terms at the time. I was simply given a direction. It was a totally natural feeling. It was as if someone had walked up to my door and said, 'Hi. My name is so-and-so. I'm selling books.' It didn't seem like anything out of the ordinary."

She felt that this was the beginning of a "waking-up" process. She was happy and excited although she missed her husband and wished he were there to share her experiences with her.

She described another experience.

> One night I was writing in my journal. I was writing about things that had happened during the day and then it was like something else occurred and I started writing in big print. And what I had written was, "All questions will be answered at the right time." And to be still and be calm, and I can't remember exactly what else at this point. But then I wrote—it's like

recognition dawned in me: "*I am* is talking to myself." And it hit me, who "I am" *is.* I deemed myself at that moment as being one who had been informed that I was a baby god. I recognized my babyhood. I was not god over anybody else. It was that I was a child god. And then I wrote again, "All questions will be answered when the time is right, no sooner, no later. Stay open, don't push, be still, be thankful, remember." And then I wrote, "Where the light touches, darkness is no more."

The Expert: We have here bizarre ideation, grandiose thoughts, delusions of reference. The patient must be placed on medication immediately and be helped to realize that she will never be able to lead a normal life. It is essential that over-stimulation be avoided. The pathology is evidently deeply rooted and the damage to her psyche is irreversible. This is a tragic case.

She now felt safe and secure and very happy.

I had been looking outside of myself all the time for direction, when I felt like I really had a direct connection to this thing that people call 'God', this thing that people say is up there, or over there, or somewhere else. I now knew that there was no separation between me and this power, this person. There was no question. It was like I had just been informed and it was the happiest news I could ever get, outside from the part about how we never die.

She said the realization of our immortality dawned on her when she was watching television.

It seemed to emanate from inside my head in message form. It was not a voice, it was more like a thought. But it was a direct communication, more understandable than a telephone call or talking face to face with someone. I was watching old newsreels, and it was of wars, you know, battles, people killing each other out on the fields. And it was making me very nervous because I was thinking, I really don't want to be watching people getting blown away. And at that point is when this came into the center of my brain, 'We never die. These are just actors. We've always been, we did not begin. The idea of a beginning and ending is something that people have made up. It is an illusion.'

And I know that this is expressed in Indian philosophy but I

> had not read any of that material at this time. I thought, 'We
> are just actors and we're playing roles.' And this made me feel
> extremely free, except that there was no one to tell it to,
> because at that point I was realistic enough to realize that other
> people would not accept what I had to say. And I felt as if we
> were all in a play. And everybody was doing this play and I was
> the only one in the audience.
>
> But then I began to get confused because I began to think that
> everybody knew they were in a play. And shortly after, I began
> to start talking to people about this, and that's when I started
> getting in big trouble.

She was exhausted from going so long without sleep and she
began to worry that she could not take care of her son. So she
called her parents and they agreed to let her stay with them for a
while. They came to pick her up.

> My son and I went back with her in her car and I was starting to
> babble. And I would see things—the lights had gotten real
> bright. All the lights, because it was at night. I saw a cross over a
> church that was lighted and it was just brighter than everything
> I'd ever seen. It was just wondrous. I just sat there going,
> "Wowww! What light!" I don't know how to explain it, but
> lights are still brighter to me. It's never gone back to the way it
> was. Colors are still brighter to me than they were before that.

Going to her parents' house turned out to be a poor idea. She
was clearly in an altered state of consciousness and this frightened her parents. "I began to get very afraid because they were
very afraid."

In her own house she felt secure but she felt so tired that she
was afraid that she was going to go to sleep and she wouldn't be
able to take care of her son. She had gotten barely any sleep in a
week. She wishes in retrospect that she had an alternative place
to go.

Psychiatric Medication

She agreed with her mother to go see a psychiatrist.

> We sat with him in this room, at a table—she was on my right,
> he was on my left—and she was telling him how my husband
> had left me, blah-blah-blah, and that I hadn't been sleeping,
> and he started mumbling. All of a sudden I couldn't under-
> stand what he said, he went into a mumble. And then I heard a
> sort of a hum start in the middle of my head. And with this

hum came an understanding—it was not words, it wasn't even a thought—but understanding that I was to get up and go out this door, turn left and go out this other door. I'd never been in the building before. But it showed me how to get out.

And I found myself standing outside on the sidewalk. And I was directed to look to my left and out across a field. I did, and my eyes landed on three crosses of a church, three big crosses that were planted in the ground. And I knew I was supposed to go there. And I started walking across the field. My mother, I heard her calling me. I wasn't going to look back, I just kept walking. And I felt her coming, and I turned and I saw her coming across. And that's when things really got interesting. I wasn't at the crosses yet, there was a highway and another field between me and the crosses. I turned around and my arm went up and pointed at her and my voice said, "Get away from me, Satan!"

It was not intentional on my part. It was as if someone had come in with me. I was not possessed, because I was conscious and I agreed with what was happening, even though it sort of puzzled me, in a way. There was nothing harmful or inherently bad about what was happening. So I consented to it. And after I said that to her I climbed over the fence and I walked across the four-lane highway, and I was aware that normally I would look to the right and left to see if there were any cars coming. But I did not turn my head to the right or the left because I was aware, I could feel, that there were no cars. Obviously there weren't: I did not get run over, nobody put on their brakes real fast or anything. I got to the crosses and then I thought, 'Now what?' And then I was directed again. I was directed to walk around the crosses three times, three crosses. Then to stop in front of the middle cross and to back up, and I felt almost as if somebody had their hands on me and was positioning me, only I didn't feel actual, physical touch. And it was like I was a spectator, watching, thinking, 'Well, okay, what's gonna happen with me now? What are you showing me?' And so my body backed up to the middle cross and my arms came out to the side and my feet went together and I was just in this pose for a few seconds. And it was almost like a grip that I couldn't break and I wasn't trying to break. But then it released and I walked down the hill a little ways and I just lay down on the grass. And I thought, 'Now I am dead.'

I didn't get to think very far because at this point here comes an ambulance driving up over the grass and up the side lane. And people were telling me to get in this vehicle. So something inside me said, 'Don't resist'. I get in. And I did resist when they started to strap me in. I didn't like that. I wasn't violent. I wasn't going to jump out of the truck or anything like that. And they took me over to the hospital, just the regular county hospital, and a doctor there talked to me.

She was in a distressed state now. And she was saying things that ordinarily she would have known to keep private. She told the doctor that there was going to be a big party and that there were going to be a lot of people there. People who had supposedly died would be there. He told her that he was going to give her some medication in the form of an injection.

The thought 'Poison' went through my head, and I did not want him to do it. I didn't know what it was he had but I knew it was not good for me. But he kept prodding me, he kept telling me, "You really need to do this," and "Look what you're doing to your mother." My mother was standing there and she was crying. At first I wanted to laugh because I thought, 'Yes, she's just playing her part. She's just being—she's just acting her part and she's doing it well.' But then I thought, 'No, she's really hurting.' I got very confused. So I finally agreed to take this shot. I forgot that it was poison. And it was Thorazine.

She went back to her mother's house with a supply of Thorazine. The effect of the Thorazine was powerful and immediate. Whereas previously all her visions had been "pure and good", now they became "distorted, terrifying".

I could smell my parents' fear. I tried to get away from their house, I tried to take my son and walk down to a bowling alley for a while, just to get away from them. And they ran out there and grabbed my son and said to come back or they were going to call the police. I thought, 'Oh, damn!' They kept thinking I was going to run away and get run over somewhere. But all I wanted was to get away from them and to be alone. I had no intention of hurting myself or my son. So I went back into the house and I was there for about three more days.

I still couldn't sleep. Mother kept insisting that I take the Thorazine pills and it was having the most horrifying effect on me. I had burning sensations all over my body. They would just come and go, just wash through me like I was on fire. I felt like I was going to explode if I moved. My parents looked all beet red to me. I was afraid they were gonna burn up. At one point I grabbed my son and threw him and me both in the shower and turned the cold water on with our clothes on because I had seen his face just go red. I had read a long time ago about spontaneous human combustion, and I think that was part of

what was coloring the hallucination. But I don't think I would
have had that hallucination without the Thorazine.

Imprisonment and Torture

Her parents tracked down her husband, who came to assist them
in taking care of her. Barbara's first thought was, 'He'll understand. He'll save me.' But Daniel had already decided that the
way to fulfill his marital responsibility was to help place her in a
mental hospital. He called an ambulance.

They tied me down to a stretcher so that I wouldn't fall out.
And my husband rode with me in the ambulance. When we got
to the hospital I was hanging onto his arm and my mother was
over filling out some forms. And I kept saying, "Let's get out of
here", because it smelled like death and fear. I mean I had
never smelled fear or death so bad as in that place. And I didn't
even know what that place was yet. And my mother had me
sign this form and I did it because my husband kept saying,
"We'll leave in a minute. We'll leave in a minute." But after
that I was in a room, my husband and my mother were gone,
and this jerk in white clothes had his hand on my knee asking
me if that bothered me. They had tricked me. My husband
betrayed me.

They took me into a ward and everything seemed strange.
Nothing was familiar except the sun, which I saw shining from
outside the window. I felt like the sun was the only friend I had.
And of course I couldn't reach the sun because it was way up
there and it was hot. And the next thing I remember is that I'm
standing in this room and there are people all over the place
looking at me. And I'm looking amongst all of them trying to
find anyone that would look like a friend.

And I saw this young man, a Mexican guy with long hair, and
I thought to myself, 'Friend'. I thought, 'Wolf brother', because
he made me think of a Native American and I just started
walking toward him. I couldn't talk. I was so terrified that I
could not talk. But I knew that he was a safe person to be with.
And I had my arm out just to touch his arm. And before I got
within three feet of him there were three attendants on top of
me. They dragged me off into another room and they gave me a
shot. I was protesting, I was screaming, I was telling them,
"Don't, don't", because I knew it was gonna be something bad.
They undid my pants and they shot me in the rear end and put
me in a room and locked the door. And I was just absolutely
terrified.

"From the drugs? Terrified of being alone?" I asked.

Both. Because I couldn't put everything together. A little while after they gave me that shot, I heard someone screaming in the hallway. I got scared, I got worried. I thought, 'Oh, God, it must be my mother. I haven't protected her.' It was just terrifying. And I could smell something and I started getting pictures in my mind of Nazi concentration camps and they were gassing people and . . .

I responded, "They are just like Nazi concentration camps. The only thing that's missing is the ovens."

Yes, I know that now. And the thing that calmed me down was that another Mexican guy came up and looked at me through the window of the door in isolation. There were a lot of Hispanic people in the hospital because this was San Antonio. He looked at me, seemed real calm. He held up a cigarette. I couldn't hear him but I could tell by his gestures that he was asking me, 'Do you want one?' I nodded and he lit it and rolled it under the door. And I started trying to calm down a little bit.

And when they finally let me out I found him and sat down beside him and just started observing everything. And that's what I spent 13 days doing, observing what was going on, what was happening. I saw them hauling people around and I saw them take people away, and forcibly inject them, and put them in isolation when they weren't doing anything to harm people. They were just frightened. And they would not let me outside. I wanted to get out, but I had no intention of escaping because there was nowhere to go.

A variety of different therapists saw her and they would ask her questions like, 'Do you hear voices?' 'What's your name?' 'How old are you?' They also kept asking her if she would leave her husband alone after she was released from the hospital. "Because my mother did not want me to bother him and he did not want me to bother him. He never would talk with me when I was in the hospital." The doctor seemed relieved when Barbara told him that she would leave her husband alone.

After 13 days she got out of the hospital. This was in large part because "I learned to shut up about what was happening and act normal for them. And so I had enough of the proper answers, to the point where the woman was willing to think about it." The doctor finally signed her release form.

When she got out of the hospital she drove to her husband's house. She now knew where he was staying. I asked her what she wanted from her husband. Barbara said that she just wanted him to talk with her, to sit down and try to "work things out". And as soon as she got to her husband's house he got scared and he called the sheriff. The sheriff said that she wasn't doing anything wrong and that there was nothing he could do. Her husband then called her mother and asked her mother to come pick her up. Her mother told her husband to bring Barbara to her mother's and father's home. At this point Daniel just took off in his truck and left.

Barbara at this point gave up all attempts to communicate with her husband. She got back in her truck and drove home. When she got to her home she felt relieved and decided she was going to get a good night's sleep. But as soon as she got out of the truck she noticed that the sheriff's deputy's truck was behind her. And then she noticed her mother's car driving up. And they said to her, "We need to take you for a psychiatric examination." She said, "Look. I want to go in and rest." A woman who was living in her apartment building came out and said, "Let her stay here. We'll take care of her, she's all right." But Barbara's mother was emphatic about her having a psychiatric examination. The sheriff's deputy assured her it would only take 30 minutes. So to please them and avoid an argument she agreed to go.

Although she was exhausted and distressed she tried to appear as 'normal' as possible. She lost the battle when she heard a child in the next room scream.

> I knew not to run to the child, because I had made that mistake in the first place, in the first hospital. I had heard a baby cry, and not realizing it was a nursery my instinct was to go to it. And I had gotten dragged down by a couple of cops. But in this case I held my ground, but my head moved. I jerked and my eyes got wide, and I looked toward the sound.
> "Does that upset you?" the psychiatrist asked.
> And I said, "Well, yes."
> And he said, "Well, he's just getting a stitch in his finger."

I responded, "The psychiatrist evidently regarded the fact that you were upset by the pain of another human being as a symptom that you were schizophrenic."

"Yes," she said. "And also I was getting confused because I had still not slept."

Before she knew it she was in Austin State Hospital. They gave her an injection of psychiatric drugs. When she woke up she was in the day room of a huge ward. No one had offered her a bed and

she had had no food. They put her on Navane, another neuroleptic. Once again the drugs had a devastating effect on her. "My
eyes rolled up, I'd stiffen up all over, I'd be sitting there and fall
over to one side. And I had to fight like hell to keep from
drooling. I took the drugs because I knew that if I didn't take it
they would give it to me in the form of an injection."

The drugs made her extremely restless. "I would be pacing. Or
I would sit down but I could only sit down for a few seconds, then
I'd have to jump again and keep moving."

"And you hadn't had the restlessness before the drugs, when
you were in your house, unable to sleep?" I asked.

"No, I didn't feel I had to pace. I just couldn't sleep."

Toward the end of her stay in the hospital she asked the male
nurse, who was very sympathetic, "Let me just take half of it this
time. Okay?"

"He agreed. And I took half of it and I felt myself come down
to ground. I saw things totally more clearly than I had in a long
time."

After 15 days she requested a court hearing to be released.
When she met her attorney he told her that he thought she was
very sick and she should stay in the hospital. Barbara said to him,
"Listen. If you don't believe in me you're not going to defend me.
I'll talk to the judge myself. I'm not going to stay in the hospital.
It's not a good thing."

And surprisingly he said, "Well, just a minute." And he went
in and talked to the judge, and came back. And he said, "Okay,
you're released. But you have to go back to sign out."

Barbara called a friend of hers who lived in Austin and she
went to stay at her house for a few days. After several days she
met with her husband's lawyer and signed the divorce papers.
She moved to a new house several miles from the one where she
had lived with her husband. She stopped taking psychiatric drugs
but went to her family doctor and got a prescription again for
Ativan, which helped calm her and made it easier for her to sleep.
She took care of her son and started working cleaning houses to
make extra money. This was in 1984.

For the next three years things went smoothly, until 1987,
when she ended up back in the hospital again. She attributed this
to a combination of feeling lonely and of being pressured by her
parents to go out and get a job. At that point she was no longer
working. "And I was still trying to be a mother. That was my
main job in my mind."

Her parents kept saying, "We can't give you any more money.

We're running out of money. We're not going to live forever." An additional factor causing her to become distressed was that she stopped taking Ativan abruptly, and she began to experience withdrawal symptoms. Her mother came to visit her. She tried to communicate some of the unusual experiences she was having, experiences of being in touch with two realities at the same time. "I was trying to draw them a picture in the air, like, I'm in the doorway: 'You're on one side, the other side is over here, I have access to both.' For some reason I was thinking, it was wishful thinking, 'They're gonna understand this. They'll see.' And they didn't."

They put her back in San Antonio State Hospital. Once again she was forced to take neuroleptic drugs.

> Oh, God, it wreaked havoc with me! I mean, it would make my breathing stop. I would be sitting there and my head would just twirl around, like when you're doing neck exercises. It would just do that every once in a while. I would be shuffling slowly down a hallway and my feet would just stop. And I'd have to just stand there and I'd get embarrassed and just kind of lean on the wall because my feet wouldn't move.
>
> And again I couldn't sleep. They put me in the observation room, and the attendants there were horrible. They had a card table set up against the wall right outside my door. And all night long they were playing cards and banging that damn table on the wall and then wondering why I couldn't get any rest. And also every time I'd start to doze off my breathing would stop and I'd get scared and it would jerk me back. And I'd feel this restlessness from the drugs and I'd be walking around the day room all day long.
>
> Anyway, I was there about 45 days. I had given up. I said, 'To hell with everybody. They don't give a shit. I'll just die.' But I couldn't die. I didn't die. A guy came along, a patient, an alcohol abuser who had attempted suicide, and he offered a caring hand.

Release and Rehabilitation

Barbara became romantically involved with him. She felt loved. Her will to live revived. "One attendant told my boyfriend that he ought to forget me because I was completely gone. But he disregarded them. I became alive again because it made me believe that somebody could care, somebody actually *did*. It got me out of the hospital."

The Expert: The patient is too severely damaged to manage the demands of an intimate relationship.

After 45 days she and her boyfriend were both released on a furlough for a week. Barbara took him to her house with her. "I began to have my own good visions again in spite of the drugs. And I knew there was no way I was going back."

This time her mother was sympathetic to her because she had finally come to realize how destructive the hospitals were. So her mother helped to arrange for her to sign the forms that would make her release from the hospital legal. She signed the forms and was released. She agreed with their request that she go to a community clinic. She agreed to take Lithium. She said the Lithium made her feel nauseated and that it kept her in "a kind of a fog". It was not as unpleasant as the neuroleptics, but "nevertheless I did not want it because I knew it would cause birth defects and all that kind of stuff." She was living with her boyfriend at the time.

She found a psychiatrist there who consented to her request not to take Lithium. He agreed to give her a prescription for Ativan, which she took at a very low dose to help her to sleep.

She has not taken any neuroleptic drugs or Lithium since her hospitalization in 1987. According to the mental health establishment, she ought to be experiencing psychotic episodes because she, ostensibly, has a chronic mental illness. Barbara quoted for me from records that she had procured from the hospital where she was incarcerated in March 1987:

> The patient needs to be made fully aware of the importance of the chemotherapy program and clinic appointments if she is to maintain her stability while out in the community. This is the second admission [to this particular hospital] for this 32-year-old Anglo female. It appears that the patient did not fully comply with the chemotherapy program and has now regressed to the point that restabilization is needed and, as mentioned above, the importance of adhering to the chemotherapy should be emphasized to her if she is to do well in the community.

Barbara said, "They're blaming it on the fact that I wasn't taking this garbage. You know, how did I manage without it for three years then?"

Barbara was told that if she was not to decompensate she would need to go to a day treatment center. She agreed.

"Did you find it demeaning?" I asked.

Hell, yes! They kept everybody like children. And when I tried
to tell different people that were in there, different clients,
about my experience and that I didn't take drugs, they would
tell me, in front of these people, that I was different, that I was
not as sick as they were.

And I finally had to get out of that place altogether because I
couldn't get anywhere with the clients. They were totally
brainwashed by the staff, totally dependent on being told what
to do by the staff. The staff had them working in their
workshop, their wood shop, for eight cents a piece on little
things that they'd do, or putting brass parts together and stuff.
And they encouraged people to take their 'medications' all the
time. I mean, people over there, a lot of them, would go to sleep
during group therapy or whatever. They were just as drugged
out as they were in the hospitals.

She left the day treatment center. She returned to her home
where she was living with her boyfriend. She stayed "in visions"
for three months. But this time she was prudent enough not to
tell anyone.

I felt a connectedness with every other living being, with
everything. And I felt at times I had the ability to know what
people were feeling. It wasn't merely a thought of my
relatedness to other beings, it was an experiential knowledge.
In normal consciousness for me there is such a thing as a
stranger, there is such a thing as a person that I'm not related to
in any way. But in this other consciousness I am very well
aware of my relatedness to people just as I normally am with
my own brother, my mother or my father. I felt very good.

The relationship with her boyfriend ended several months
later. He frequently drank too much and he would become
verbally abusive with Barbara. She found a therapist at the
community center who was more or less on her wavelength. He
treated her with respect and did not regard her as a 'mental
patient'. Barbara still takes Ativan to help her when she's feeling
anxious, but she's reduced her dosage of the drug and intends to
give it up altogether. It was Barbara who initiated the separation
from her boyfriend.

I noted that she was being the assertive one this time.

She responded, "Yes. I didn't want to. It hurt. It felt like I was
throwing a puppy dog out into the wild, because that's the way he
came on to me: 'Please don't do this. I love you, I love you, I love
you'. But he refused to make any effort to control his drinking."

Barbara is now a mother. She dates men occasionally, she

keeps a journal and she has started an organization opposed to psychiatric abuse. She is a volunteer in the Austin State Hospital psychiatric ward one day a week. She has been experiencing tension with the staff there. "I'm not supposed to be there as a volunteer. I'm not supposed to be able to do these things. I'm supposed to be out on psychiatric drugs somewhere being the good patient."

I asked her what she thought enabled her to resist being inducted into the career of a mental patient. Why did she not become indoctrinated like the others? In other words, why was she able to go through madness and to go through the indoctrination and invalidation process of the psychiatric establishment and emerge with the will to fight?

> I could not forget my original visions and the reality of them. I knew that what was going on was valid for me. They had made me doubt it to a point, but not very much. And once I got out of the hospital the first time I began to go into the libraries and start looking for verification. I remember going into a bookstore and I started grabbing books like it was somebody telling me, 'Pick up this one. Pick up this one. Pick up this one'. And one of them that I picked up was *The Politics of Experience,* by R.D. Laing. And the effect it had on me was, 'My God! This person knows exactly what I'm going through and he's a psychiatrist. So there's hope. And this shows me there's somebody alive that knows what I'm talking about'. Because before that all I had read was Edgar Cayce who died in 1945. I found another book, Carl Jung's *Man and His Symbols.* And I saw people writing about experiences that I had. And it's not in a 'mentally ill' context. So the self-doubt as far as my visions were concerned never had a chance to get hold of me. There was a core of me that believed in myself, that they could not drug out of me.

How Barbara Beat the System

Like the expert in this chapter, most therapists would attribute Barbara's dissatisfaction in her relationships with men to an alleged defect in her psyche. The environmental factors causing the dissatisfaction would be completely overlooked. This is not to deny that Barbara may have developed, in her family of origin, self-generated patterns of behavior that limited her ability to achieve satisfaction, patterns subject to change.

She herself pointed out in our interview that when she first became involved with men she had a tendency to be submissive, to attempt to appease them. But to attribute this *habit* to a defect in her psyche is to make a metaphysical leap that is unwarranted. The assertion that she is 'mentally ill' contains two premises: 1. There has been a diminution or annulment of her worth as a human being: her psyche is defective; and 2. She has no freedom of will; her actions are 'symptoms' of 'psychopathology'.

The first premise is reflective of the contempt the experts feel for their 'patients'. There is no justification for construing an *aspiring* or struggling person as a 'damaged' person. The second premise is rendered less credible by Barbara's own actions. She transcended on her own, without the help of a therapist, a limiting pattern of behavior. In her youth she *chose* a particular strategy as a way of achieving or maintaining interpersonal intimacy. In the course of her story she *chooses* to give this strategy up. She learns to be assertive with men.

Barbara is a woman who desires to engage in mutual self-disclosure with the men in her life. This is not a symptom of pathological neediness, it is a genuine human need (albeit one not always easily fulfilled). It is a fact that men in this country are less inclined to 'open up' in this manner. It is this environmental factor that leads Barbara to experience frustration.

She risks confronting her husband Daniel, she risks asserting her independence to the man who pledged to spend his life with her, and with whom she pledged to spend her life—and she experiences the shock of her life. He flees in terror. He abandons her. One does not need to be an expert to appreciate what an excruciatingly, exquisitely painful kind of experience this is. Unfortunately, tragically, the expertise of the mental health pundits prevents them from appreciating this. Instead they viewed her distress not as a natural response to betrayal and abandonment but as a symptom of a chronic mental illness, as a sign that she is mentally defective. What could be more damning proof that the mental health establishment trains therapists to become emotionally discombobulated imbeciles (regardless of their IQs)?

In the period of Barbara's greatest distress she had a number of extraordinary transcendental experiences. Like mystics of all ages she experienced the unity of the human species. Whether one grants validity to the 'visions' she had or not, they were undoubtedly extraordinary, vivid, colorful, ecstatic. They added richness to her life. They gave her confidence that there was an absolute, a Reality, beyond this world of appearances—a Reality

(God) that endowed human life in general, and her life in particular, with meaning.

This domain of experience is proclaimed off-limits by the mental health establishment. The experts have only one way of viewing these experiences: as signs of mental illnesses, evidently due to ego damage or to defective genes. Anyone who thinks differently is obviously naively romanticizing mental illness. It must be emphasized here: it was Barbara's trust in the authenticity of her visions that enabled her to resist being inducted into the role of a chronic mental patient.

CHAPTER SIX

Angela's Story

Angela's story begins in November 1976. She was a housewife and mother of two young boys. Her husband earned a living as a bus driver. She now believes that she was then undergoing a process of spiritual transformation. Some of the time she was disoriented, which led her concerned family to take her to the psychiatric clinic in search of help. The mental health experts believed that Angela was 'mentally ill', that she suffered from 'paranoid schizophrenia'. The more she tried to convince them of the validity of her perceptions the more certain they were that her experiences were the product of a defective psyche. Her attempts to persuade them were viewed as *further* evidence of her illness, of what they term 'denial', which is a pathological refusal to accept that one is mentally ill, in other words psychologically defective.

Only a severely damaged person would refuse to accept that she was defective when the mental-health experts were convinced that she was defective. She realized the obstacles she faced: that the version of reality that they had been indoctrinated to accept as absolute did not permit them to acknowledge the truth of her reality. Even if there were a tacit recognition at times of the validity of her insights they could not acknowledge that fact and remain in the system; her perceptions had to be classified as 'delusional thinking'.

Mystical Experiences

Angela had given some thought to the question of whether she wanted to tell me, Dr. Farber, another doctor of psychology, her story. A critical factor in her decision to go forward was the fact that my first name is 'Seth'. Since 1978 Angela had been studying the work of a medium named Jane Roberts who channelled the ideas of an allegedly disincarnate philosopher who called himself 'Seth'. (Seth was or is a philosopher in the pragmatic idealist tradition who believes that individuals create their own reality. Jane Roberts's books are available in most bookstores. Jane was never sure if 'Seth' was an actual entity or a facet of her sub-conscious or supra-conscious mind. She disregarded the mental health experts who told her that she had a 'schizoid personality disorder' and was manufacturing the Seth material in order to manipulate her husband, Rob. Angela's husband's name, incidentally, is also Rob.)

In November of 1976 Angela felt that she had entered "the universal mind". "I had a sudden awareness that we were all part of God, that we were never externalized, that we are still part of him."

Angela had a Roman Catholic background and she had recently been studying the works of Edgar Cayce but this was the first time she had had such a profound spiritual experience. Previously she had thought of God as being outside and apart from human beings. She had read mystics but her understanding was merely intellectual. "But with that first experience it just all clicked."

> And I had a million questions and every time I formulated a question the answer came right on top of it—in non-verbal terms. But it was such a mind-expanding experience that I didn't know what had happened to me. In fact I actually thought that I must have died, that I must be in some sort of an afterlife . . . because my perceptions were so different. Everything around me had not just its own meaning but meanings going back in time. There were connections with things, like an invention or something, I would be instantly connected with the inventor. For example, the sofa would make me feel connected with the craftsman who made it, the designer of the fabric—a multitude of people connected with just that one piece of furniture. I was reading psychology and I really felt I saw Freud, I saw Jung. Freud was angry at modern psychiatry. Jung led me to a rational explanation of my experiences.

She was communing with their spirits.

The Expert: The patient is schizophrenic. She confuses her inner fantasy world with reality. The primary process material has erupted and has impeded the functioning of her ego skills, in particular her ability to recognize and adapt to the real world. The sense of grandiosity is a compensation for the low sense of self-esteem she feels as a result of the damage to her ego evidently experienced at an early stage of her development as a child.

The experience was ecstatic but it was confusing, overwhelming. "I wouldn't be able to focus on what I was doing. If I went to get a meal together I'd be talking to the lettuce, I'd be talking to the tomatoes, while making a salad. . . . I felt there was communication going on between myself and my environment. There was consciousness in everything."

Alarmed Friends and Family

I asked her if this was distressing in any way. "It was wonderful! It was as if I had just gotten the code to the universe or something. The only source of distress came from people around me who were not very tolerant of my behavior."

I asked her if she thought she was a danger to herself or anyone else in this unusual state of consciousness. She said she was not but that her friends and family became frightened that she would try to kill herself. They reasoned that since she thought she was dead she would try to dispose of her body.

To make things worse for her friends she did not want to go to sleep—she felt so elated. Also she figured that since she was dead she did not need sleep or food. Nevertheless she got a minimal amount of sleep and she continued to eat. She continued to fulfill her material responsibilities though it was difficult at times. "I was seeing my own kids' past lives and future when I was trying just to give them a bath." Love-making with her husband was more intense and enjoyable than usual. She could not understand her husband's need for rest.

Her unusual behavior fuelled the fears of her family and friends. Her friend Colleen, who came to the interview with Angela, was not frightened. "I knew she was going through an altered state of consciousness and would never hurt anyone." Angela was babysitting for Colleen's son when Colleen got a phone call at work from a mutual friend who said, "Angie thinks she's dead. So maybe she'll try to kill the children." Colleen was alarmed at first but when she got home she was relieved. "She was very loving and caring. The fact that she thought she was dead did not change that. Besides the children were evidently not frightened by her so why should I worry?"

Angela's husband took her to the emergency room at the hospital. "Nobody asked me what I was experiencing. That's what really got me. I mean, my husband told them I was behaving bizarrely and that was enough. And I was frank with them. I said, 'Oh, well, I'm in touch with Freud and Jung and this one and that one.'"

The Expert: Clearly a deeply disturbed patient. Characterolog-
                 ical defenses prevent her from acknowledg-
                 ing that she is mentally ill, out of touch with
                 reality. An underlying schizoid personality
                 disorder prevents her from accepting the di-
                 agnosis, prevents her from realizing the es-
                 sential defect in her self. Delusions of
                 reference are a compensation for the gnaw-
                 ing sense of inadequacy this emotionally
                 damaged woman feels. This is a tragic case.
                 The prognosis is poor.

Incarceration and Drugs

Sitting in the emergency room evoked a variety of emotions. It was the same hospital she had been born in. She inferred from this that she was back there to be born again. "And they sat me in a little room and there was a little button on the wall that said, 'Nurse'. And I thought if I pressed that button I was going to wind up back in an infant's body upstairs in the nursery. So I was a little confused."

She wanted to leave.

> You know, I was in a state of mind where I was really sensitive to the moods of people around me. And in that state of mind, to be brought to a psychiatric emergency room where you have so many people who are absolutely terrified. . . . Some people had been picked up by the cops for one reason or another. Some people were off the streets who don't know where their next meal was coming from and the only way they know to get another meal and a roof over their heads is to get themselves into the psychiatric ward. There was a lot of fear there and I picked up on that.

She had felt no fear before. She was confused, she had trouble making sense of what was happening, but she felt a state of well-being—at best, of euphoria. Now she was terrified. She tried several times to leave but the guards stopped her. I asked her if she had displayed any violence and she said that she had not. I asked her if she thought she would do something to harm herself. She responded that she felt, to the contrary, that she was trying to protect herself by getting out of there as quickly as possible. She was strapped down against her will on a bed and given an injection of a psychiatric drug ('medication') to make her comply.

When she woke up she was in the psychiatric ward. "I thought that the hospital was Hell. I thought I had died and this was the afterlife and now this was Hell. You know, the people were walking around like zombies. There was no appearance of their being alive. Only the staff were real and they don't even talk to you! Or they talk down to you, or they tell you to stay in your room."

She thinks it euphemistic to call psychiatric drugs medication. "They knock you out. They cause aches and pains all through your body. They make you apathetic. They stop the whole spiritual transformation process. It's like putting molasses in your brain. You can't even concentrate enough to read." She took the drugs reluctantly, after being told she would not be released unless she complied.

The psychiatrists told her husband that she was mentally ill but they were not sure what particular illness she had. (After her second breakdown 10 months later, her husband was told that she had been diagnosed as a paranoid schizophrenic.) They told her husband that she would never be normal again and that she had a disease like diabetes that would require her to take medication for the rest of her life. She was told a few weeks later, before they discharged her, that she was severely mentally ill. She was very discouraged.

> There's nothing more depressing than having somebody tell you your brain isn't working right. They kept telling me, 'You can't do all the things you're doing. You have to draw limits for yourself, you have to be reasonable.' They wanted to limit me to a mediocre existence. They said, 'You have to stay on the drugs. We realize that you may not be able to do all you did before you went on them, but this is best. You'll at least be able to function as a normal human being'.

"How horrible!" I responded.

"Damn! I don't want to function as a normal human being. I feel I have a talent that is a superior talent. But in their eyes that means I have 'delusions of grandeur'. . . . Oh yes, and they warned me to stay away from anything spiritual. That was a grave danger in their eyes. And I should not read the Bible either."

She wished that she had someone to talk to at that time,

someone to explain to her that she was undergoing a process of spiritual transformation instead of interpreting her experience as a pathological process. She felt none of the mental-health workers really listened to her.

> They never asked me what my problems were when I went in. They never asked me, you know, the kind of things that I was thinking and they would not have understood it if I had told them. . . . I would have liked to avoid the confusion I suffered for so many years because of the psychiatrists telling me that something was pathological that I knew to be right for me.

She stayed on the drugs for three months after she was released. Why? "Because I was scared. Because they didn't know what to do and this is what the doctors said. And we put an awful lot of faith in doctors. And over the years I've come to realize that they're just human beings like the rest of us, and many of them don't know what they're doing."

Spiritual Messages

When she stopped taking the drugs her life became more interesting again. She became involved in a spiritual study group where they accepted it as positive to communicate with spirits. At this point she was not hearing voices but rather "words would pop out" at her when she was reading something. That is, she would look at a page of text and certain words on the page would stand out in such a way that they constituted a sentence that was not in the text *per se.* "It was a training thing for my kids. And it said, 'This is to be a series of lessons especially designed to help you grow.' They were there in front of me, not in that order."

Later she got a message from the *TV Guide.*

> And the fact that it was the *TV Guide*—that was a pun on spirit guide. In our spiritual study group we had been talking about explorers and people who break new ground. They had this one particular article called "Columbus on the Couch". I rearranged the article, substituting my name for 'Columbus'. I did it subconsciously. I brought it out the way I was seeing it. It was an exact biography of myself. One of the things that stands out in my mind was that he was the oldest child and took responsibility for the welfare of his siblings. It paralleled my life exactly. And then it talked about exploring and getting people to back you up. And one of the lines was, "Can we now label Christopher Columbus pathologically persistent?"

"You know," I responded, "any kind of new endeavor, any kind of heroic venture can be seen and is inclined to be seen by the mental health experts as a symptom of pathology."

She showed me the article. Here are some excerpts.

> As the mists of ignorance are lifting, Columbus [Angela] is ready. Great discoveries so often result from a serious combination of ignorance and insight, persistence and pure luck.
>
> The quest consumes him [her]. Desperate for firm support, he [she] gets but slight encouragement. When questioned closely about his [her] objectives, she cannot always stay calm, and he [she] slips easily into vagueness and inconsistency. He [she] speaks of a providential mission and hears himself [herself] mocked and derided for pursuing a grand illusion. But on he [she] plods, he [she] waits, he [she] persists!
>
> Should we not be at least mildly suspicious of a man [woman] whose egocentricity and sense of mission override all doubts and extinguish self-criticism? Maybe so, but then substitute 'dogged determination' for 'sense of mission' and much of the apparent obsessive-compulsiveness fades. Can we now label Columbus [Angela] as pathologically persistent?
>
> Sound motives must be accompanied by reasonable objectives. Is Columbus [Angela] vulnerable here? Is he [she] taking too great a leap for mankind? Not at all. A revolution in thought is underway. Scientific minds are beginning to concede. The time is ripe, the age of exploration is clearly underway. If he [she] hesitates, he [she] knows well, others will not. The fact that he [she] is largely self-taught will only add lustre to his [her] achievements.
>
> Maybe we accept, all too readily, contemporary characterizations, forgetting how often the man [woman] of vision is derided for daring to think the unthinkable. Columbus [Angela] himself [herself] lamented the fact that everyone "to whom I spoke of this enterprise thought it was mere jest".
>
> Exceptional men [women] have problems being accepted.

"I took this article to my psychologist. It broke through a lot of his barriers. Of course I had had him for several years at that point and he had come to trust me."

She had a number of psychic experiences.

> We had this girl living in our house as a boarder for a while. She now calls my husband and me 'Dad' and 'Mom'. We were sitting in my living room one night and all of a sudden I saw this person standing behind her. And I knew it was an apparition because there was nobody there. And I described it to her thinking it was somebody from the past she had known.

And she said she didn't know anybody who fit this description. And he looked down at her, smiled, looked up at me, smiled, and faded out. Well, she moved out of her house into her first apartment of her own about two months after that. And she met the guy who lived upstairs from her. And that was the guy I described, and that was the guy that she married. And both of us realized he fit the description I had given her.

And another thing, he couldn't decide at first whether to make a commitment and I told her he's going to wind up going to Boston. When he comes back from Boston he'll be ready for a commitment. Now at the time he wasn't planning on going to Boston at all, he was making plans to go to Florida. He wound up going to Boston, stayed there for about a month, came back, and they got married a month later. She's 28 now and they have three children. So there are a lot of people in my immediate circle that know I have abilities that others just don't have. My kids are convinced at this point.

Her family was worried about her unusual experiences so they took her to the emergency room for an evaluation. She went willingly because she thought that she would be able to educate the mental health workers. "I thought I had enough understanding now that I could convince the psychiatrists that what was happening was not pathological. I was wrong."

I remarked that I had observed that a lot of people go back to mental hospitals hoping to get validation from psychiatrists. "It's like wanting to convince your mother or father that something you believe is true."

She said, "Because it's the psychiatrist that has invalidated the experience and it's the psychiatrist that has the *power* to invalidate. Therefore it follows that they would have the power to validate the event. But you're not about to get that from a psychiatrist! You have to come to believe in yourself despite all opposition."

When they released her from the hospital she stopped taking her 'medicine'. Once again I noted that the only really distressing experiences she described seemed to be in the hospital. She said the only other distressing experiences were related to the unexpected deaths of friends. She continued to have unusual experiences. One time she was sitting in her therapist's office and she saw a friend of hers in the room with her. This friend who had cancer appeared as six inches high and was sitting up on a bookshelf. Angela told her therapist who responded, "Why do you feel you need your friend here at this time?" The therapist was implying that Angela hallucinated her friend's presence because of a pathological need.

> And meantime my friend Dolly—everybody called her 'Crazy Dolly' because of her far-out ideas—kept making jokes. Dolly always hated psychiatrists. She said to me, "You see, I'm not afraid of shrinks any more", and it was a pun, of course, because she was six inches tall. As soon as I got home I got a call from Dolly's daughter-in-law that she had passed away at the time I was in my therapist's office. I got hysterical. I don't know why I was so hysterical. Part of it was grief over my friend's death. But it was also, you know, maybe they still don't believe me. Then I called my therapist and told her.

"Did you break through her barriers?" I asked.

> I did break through her barriers. I really did. . . . A couple of sessions after that I went into therapy and she had a poster on her wall of two seagulls flying and it said, "They can because they think they can", and I said to her, "Rachel, I believe I can talk to spirits. Is it true that I can because I think I can?" And she didn't know what to say.

Shortly after that another friend of Angela's died in a fire. That friend spoke Spanish, which Angela did not understand. But her therapist spoke Spanish. "A couple of sessions after my friend's death I started delivering messages in Spanish to my Spanish-speaking therapist. She was shocked."

"Did she acknowledge that you had psychic abilities?"

"She could not acknowledge it to me. You see, from the perspective of what they consider reality, this is 'delusional thinking.'"

"This must have created a state of cognitive dissonance. How did she handle it?"

"She left. I think she believed me. But I don't think she could handle it and keep her job. You see this is not part of their training. It's not acceptable. You cannot think this if you're a therapist treating a client."

Back Inside

Angela went back into the mental hospital five more times. Why?

"Pathological persistence, probably."

"You think it was a desire to convince them each time?"

"Yes. A big part of it was."

"Did you?"

"You can't penetrate their walls. They have walls built around them."

"They were all in unison telling you that your experiences were signs of mental illness?"

"Oh yeah. Definitely. . . . I was telling people, 'Gee, you know, they're telling me this is a disease. If it's a disease, this is the one I want to have.'"

"Was there anything therapeutic that happened to you in the hospital?"

"I met other patients. And then it got to a point where I felt as if I was being led in, just to make certain connections with people who I would meet on the inside."

One of the times she ended up back in the hospital because she had a fight with her husband.

> I was furious at him for something. He was blaming it on my so-called illness. I was just damn mad about something! I don't even remember what it was. So he said, "Come on, let's go see the doctor. Let's get you some medication." So I figured, "Okay, I'll go to psych ER, I'll talk to them, I'll be calm, I'll explain that he is the problem, not any mysterious mental illness. And then I'll be out of there." Well they had me and him waiting in this room for about an hour. And he said to me, "You're not going home unless you take your medication." I go so angry I threw the cup of coffee right over his shoulder. I was careful not to throw it on him because it was hot. But the psychiatrists concluded that that action was a sign that I was "violent and a danger to others", and I was in again.

Angela has not been in a mental hospital as a patient for five years. After the first breakdown she was on the drugs for three months. Since then she has never taken them for more than a brief period of time.

> If I listened to them and stayed on the drugs I'd probably be living on the street now. I can't cope on those drugs. They just make me confused and scared. My husband would have divorced me. And then they would have said that mental illness was the cause of my problems. When the truth is their treatment would have been the cause of my problems, as it is the cause of the problems of the people who accept their propaganda. I look at myself as privileged to have had the experiences I had, the experiences they call pathology.

Sunset was approaching and it was time to prepare to end our talk but Angela had one more experience she wanted to relate.

Her cousin Edward had a brain tumor since he was five. One day when Edward was 22 she saw him—and felt his presence—in her living room. He was singing

> "You'll Never Walk Alone." And an overlap of this was a voice saying, "If young men must die, how much better this way than in another war." And I called the emergency room and I told them I was scared because I thought Edward was going to die. And the next day he died. And my son Robby came to me and he said, "Mom, you better sit down." And I said, "Robby, I know what you are going to say. Just look what I wrote in my diary last night." A few weeks later my kids were chiding me about some of my experiences when I suddenly surprised them by a bout of laughter. I laughed because I heard Edward singing the Mr. Ed theme song with appropriate changes: "A corpse is a corpse, of course, of course. And no one can talk to a corpse of course. That is, of course, unless the corpse is the famous Mr. Ed." You know he had a sense of humor like that. I went to the emergency room after he died.

"Did they realize you had had a precognition?"

"They must have. But they did not want to admit it."

"So you've changed them?"

"Individuals I've changed over time. But then what can they do? The system will not permit them to acknowledge that what they call our pathology is really illumination."

A Well-Adjusted Schizophrenic

Angela's experience of the universe was radically different from that of the mental health experts. Hers was a cosmos peopled by spirits and disclosing continuously unexpected sources of meaning, a universe open to divine revelation. Their universe was the rationalized, bureaucratized world order described by Max Weber: the world is a machine governed by impersonal laws, conforming to the norms of a positivist science. The major premise underlying this conception of the world is, as Weber put it, that "there are no mysterious incalculable forces that come into play, but rather one can in principle master all things by calculations."[1] The mental health experts live comfortably in a world that has become "disenchanted" (to borrow Weber's

---

[1]Hans Gerth and C. Wright Mills, Max Weber: *Essays in Sociology* (New York: Oxford University Press, 1958), 139

phrase again) and they regard any attempt to reverse the process of disenchantment, that is to say any attempt to participate in a re-enchantment of the world, as a threat.

What the experts viewed as the symptoms of a disease process Angela understood retrospectively (and, to a limited extent, at the time) as a process of spiritual transformation, of consciousness expansion. It was an unsettling process but it would have been far less so had she received support and guidance rather than the psychological and pharmacological abuse that was termed 'psychiatric treatment'. She derived emotional support from individuals within the system who were able to appreciate her as a person and even at times to confirm the validity of her perceptions. But two points need to be made here. In the first place, the 'professional' training of these therapists in no way aided but only impeded their ability to respond to her as a person and to recognize her gifts. Secondly, to earn this recognition required enormous persistence on her part which reflected an extraordinary strength of will.

It was these qualities that made her exceptional compared to the hundreds of thousands who give up and accept their assigned parts—the chronically mentally ill—in the drama scripted by the mental health experts. That is to say that if there is such a thing as a schizophrenic, Angela is one. She manifested all the symptoms. She was *not* misdiagnosed. She is today in their terms a well-functioning, well-adjusted schizophrenic. But, of course, this is a contradiction in terms and only goes to reveal the utter inadequacy of the dominant paradigm in psychology.

As early as 1964 R.D. Laing had described 'schizophrenics' (individuals today are more likely to be diagnosed as 'manic-depressive') as individuals who were exploring the inner world where psychiatrists fear to tread. He wrote: "Perhaps we will learn to accord to the so-called schizophrenics who have come back to us, perhaps after years, no less respect than the often no less lost explorers of the Renaissance. If the human race survives, future men will, I suspect, look on our enlightened epic as a veritable Age of Darkness. . . . They will see that what we call 'schizophrenia' was one of the forms in which, often through quite ordinary people, the light began to break through the cracks in our all-too-closed minds."[2]

Several months ago Angela wrote about her experience:

[2]R.D. Laing, *The Politics of Experience* (New York: Pantheon, 1968), 129

Thomas Szasz once said that if you talk to God—that's called prayer. If God talks to you—that's called schizophrenia.

Well, something was talking to me, explaining things to me, scaring the hell out of me at times, but over all, filling me with a sense of wonder and awe such as I had never before experienced.

I couldn't turn it off. I wouldn't sleep because I thought I might miss something important, and within a few days, I was so disoriented I didn't know who my kids were, even my own name.

. . . Everywhere you look—through any media form—the world is personally interactive. Psychiatrists call that referential thinking.

The idea that there is a cosmic intelligence that communicates to individuals through the universe was held for many centuries before the disenchantment of the world began. Carl Jung revived this concept with his theory of synchronicity. The theory posits that uncanny and meaningful coincidences occur and that they are an expression of an underlying ordering force in the universe. These synchronicities may be said to constitute a divine script.

Angela had been diagnosed as a 'paranoid schizophrenic'. R.D. Laing was viewed by the Establishment as an extremist who 'romanticized' the suffering of the 'mentally ill'. The mental health experts have succeeded in de-romanticizing virtually every dimension of human experience, leaving us with a universe denuded of meaning, bereft of poetry, a lifeless machine. They claim that this is the path to safety: outside of their jurisdiction lies madness, terror, chaos. Their alternative is a lifetime on mind-disabling psychiatric drugs, a self-concept as a flawed individual, and a disenchanted world. They speak with the authority of Medicine, of Science.

Those of us with a grander vision of human possibility will refuse to sanction as reality this vision of a soulless universe that has cast a spell upon the collective imagination of humanity. We refuse to collaborate in this process: "the disenchantment of the world and its transformation into a causal mechanism".[3] We will protest, we will fight—in the name of the Imagination, in the name of Love, in the name of God, in the name of Madness.

[3]Gerth and Mills, *op. cit.,* 350

CHAPTER SEVEN

David's Story

David Oaks is the editor of the magazine *Dendron,* a forum for individuals in the mental patient liberation movement. He has been active in that movement since his senior year at Harvard in 1977. He makes a living as a peace and environmental activist. Despite five incarcerations in mental hospitals due to emotional distress during the time when he attended Harvard, he graduated *cum laude* in the typical four-year period. He was given various diagnoses such as 'schizophrenic' and 'manic-depressive'. In other words David is supposed to be 'chronically mentally ill' and able to function at a minimal level with the help of 'medication'. He has taken no psychiatric drugs, nor been in a mental hospital, since 1977.

A Difficult Transition

Going to Harvard represented a major transition for David. "I came from a working-class background. I went to an all-male, Jesuit high school and then went with a union scholarship to Harvard." Harvard represented *making it.* His parents wanted to help him 'mainstream'.

The summer before he started school he had two part-time jobs as an office worker. "When I got to Harvard that freshman year I was totally exhausted and out of it. And I didn't have clothes that made me feel as if I fit in. I had these clothes that were really awkward."

The culture was different from the one he was used to. His high school was competitive in an overt and obvious way. "People were very into competition and cutting each other down. Brutal insult kind of thing." David's father worked as a clerk for Penn Central Railroad. He had little formal education but he spent much of his time reading. David's mother was a housewife who also loved the written word. They lived in Chicago.

The Jesuit high school he went to was preparing students for college. It was oppressively all-male. It was intellectually stimulating, highly structured, competitive but in a way that was familiar to him. "Harvard is an elitist place. It is extremely competitive and it puts you down emotionally." The students there *seemed* very fraternal, "comfortable" with themselves. "But deep down there was a kind of elitist competitiveness."

Would he make it? Would he fit in? "I came from a working-class background and I was going to Harvard and people don't understand how that kind of thing affects you to the very cells of your being."

He had the opportunity to be socially confirmed and credentialed as being a member of 'the best and brightest'. "Harvard mainly offers a mentality of elitism. Your ego gets pumped up. But in this society where we are beaten down so much that's quite a commodity to get, isn't it? They're pumping air into people's heads there."

But the opportunity to succeed was paired with the omnipresent threat of failure, a threat that transformed David's sojourn at Harvard into a prolonged identity crisis and that explained in part the moments of acute distress that led to his incarcerations in mental hospitals.

Going to Harvard also represented to David the opportunity of transcending the limitations of the environment he grew up in and that had influenced him to some extent. It was a first step to becoming a leader in the movement for social change in this country. The South Side neighborhood that David grew up in was ethnic blue-collar and racist. "The Nazi party had a headquarters only about 10 blocks from my house."

He felt that he had internalized some racial animosity which he became aware of and transcended during his years at Harvard away from his old community. "Martin Luther King came to my neighborhood and he said he saw more hatred there than he did in any part of the country. I read later after I finished college that he felt almost hopeless. The only hope was if a few of the young people got out and went to college. And I thought: that's a message for me."

The threat of not making it haunted David throughout the four years he was at Harvard and the memory of it still disturbs him occasionally today, 13 years later. "I actually still have nightmares in which I'll experience this enormous, almost cloud-like, megalithic feeling of being encompassed by this intellectual womb, which I take to be Harvard. I'm in a class and I'm not prepared for an exam. I had never even gone to the classes for it. This is a common nightmare. But in mine, I am returning from a break. I can't concentrate or remember."

The pressure for David was intensified after his first hospitalization when the authorities attempted to confer upon him the degraded social identity of a person who was 'mentally ill'. In the process of climbing the mountain he slipped and risked being hurled into the abyss of non-person status ('the chronically mentally ill') from which many individuals never escape. "Always, in this nightmare, I had left Harvard, and I've flipped out, and I'm coming back to Harvard, and I'm looking at the exam, or trying to find my way around campus. I can't read. Just like the first time after I was hospitalized and I couldn't read. I can't think. And I'm trying to piece together what's happening. And it's hard and I'm making mistakes."

Religious Experiences

Harvard was an impersonal environment. "You don't have that much personal attention from people. You rarely interact with the professor. You have huge classes with sections led by graduate students who are a few years older than you."

It was not until his sophomore year that he "flipped out".

> It was strange because I began having a Christian religious-based experience and for years I had defined myself as an atheist. . . . The images and beliefs that I had learned in high school in terms of saints and the Holy Spirit . . . came flooding back and I experienced what I thought was the Holy Spirit which led me into kind of a dangerous Boston neighborhood. I had not slept in days and I was very tired and I turned into a Jesuit school and I asked to speak with a priest. He was no help. He called my friends who took me to the psychiatric unit at Stillman Infirmary, which is right in Harvard Square. . . . I saw a woman psychiatrist and I had remembered seeing a poster around Cambridge criticizing psychiatric drugs and psychiatry so I was suspicious and told her what she wanted to hear.

He was released. He went back to the dormitory but he was still in a state of distress. His distress distressed his friends, which distressed David more. His friends took him back to Stillman. One girl said as she was about to leave him at Stillman, "Dave, you're in a lot of trouble." "Those were her last words before leaving, which scared the hell out of me. Not a smart thing to tell a person—and this was my friend."

He was placed in a room. He refused to take the drugs. "I began panicking that because I had done this, gone to the priest and so forth, that Harvard was going to put me on trial, and I'd be thrown out." The element of truth in his 'delusion' was the realistic possibility of not 'making it' at Harvard, the threat of failure that haunted this working-class boy throughout his four-year initiation at Harvard.

There were positive aspects to his experience. "I felt I could see a pattern of an angel in a door and I felt the Holy Spirit had guided me." His friends had brought him the huge book, *Lives of the Saints.* "I began identifying with the saints."

He decided that he could lessen the threat of retribution by taking the drugs so he reluctantly decided to do that. He was given a combination of Thorazine and Stelazine.

> The neuroleptics made me feel like a zombie. . . . I remember my parents had flown out to see me and I tried to reassure them that I was physically okay. I started to do some push-ups. I did a few and then I began to bite my tongue. And I tried to open my mouth and I couldn't. And my whole body was in parox-ysms. My parents got a doctor and they're watching me, this total writhing thing, and they put me onto the bed. Then a whole bunch of medical personnel showed up and they admin-istered an emergency dose of some kind of real tranquilizers that put me to sleep.

He got out of Stillman about two weeks later and tried to go back to school, but he couldn't concentrate. He went home to Chicago for a few weeks. He was in an altered state of consciousness but he felt he was in a safe supportive environment and was able to enjoy many of the unusual experiences he had. "I felt a third eye in the middle of my forehead." At that time he had only passingly read the Indian literature that described the existence of a 'third eye', whose power could be developed, enabling one to attain clairvoyant vision. "It felt as if someone was trying to place a diamond in my third eye."

David felt at times that the TV was personally communicating with him. He explains this experience now as partly a self-generated attempt to compensate for the spiritual vacuity of modern society.

> In Native American cultures, in Earth-based religious cultures, people speak freely about relating directly to nature. And they believe that nature gives them messages. The belief that nature directly communicates to you is common in these Earth-based religions. We now live in an era where we are enclosed in a glass sphere, a bubble, of technology. So my way of restoring the

sense of a dialogue with my environment was believing that the
TV was personally sending messages to me.

I responded, "It could also be that you intuitively turned on
the TV or selectively attended to the sound of the TV at times
when it was saying things that were relevant to your situation.
Carl Jung documented numerous examples of this phenomenon
which he termed synchronicity. After all, why should God
restrict Himself or Herself to communication through the medium of nature?"

Some of his experiences were more distressing. His family was
supportive. His grandparents on both sides grew up in Lithuania.
David felt that Lithuania had an 'ancient' culture and belief-
system that validated the kinds of experiences that would be
viewed as symptoms of mental illnesses in our culture.

His uncle was particularly helpful. David remembered one
time he expressed to his uncle his fear that the wall in the house
would fall. His uncle pressed up against the wall and said, "Don't
worry. I'll just hold up the wall." "My uncle was actually willing
to give credence to my experience. He was very interested in ESP
and parapsychology. . . . So when he was there I was able to calm
down. Once, I stared at a TV antenna as a kind of meditation
technique to help me to focus so that I could be centered and
lucid and still be in an altered state of consciousness but not
panicking."

He described an experience with his brother that was both
reassuring and inspiring.

> I was waiting in the car. I saw my brother go into McDonald's
> and I saw this kind of macho guy walk in after him with what
> looked like a board in his hand. I felt the guy's hostility. My
> brother walked back out, cheerful and tough at the same time.
> Something about his air of independence protected him.
> Seeing my brother come out safe in the most dangerous areas I
> realized that I could also. I could walk through this wall of
> flame and if I had support I could remain calm and lucid. It
> took me a while to develop that ability but now I am capable of
> being in a so-called psychotic state without freaking out. I can
> go back and forth.

After several weeks at home life returned to normal and David
went back to school. He made up for lost time so that by the end
of the summer he was caught up with his school work.

In his junior year he started once again to have ecstatic
mystical experiences. He cultivated these states because he felt
that it was part of a process of becoming a more whole person.

He felt that he had a tendency to be too analytical, controlling, hierarchical, distancing, over-competitive, linear. He wanted to move away from a 'left-brained' dominant mode of experiencing the world, because he felt it limited his potential as a human being. He feels that Theodore Roszak's book *The Making of the Counterculture* explains his attitude then: creativity transcending the technocratic state.

At that time he was appointed publisher of a poetry magazine for Harvard students called *padam aram,* which means 'stairway to heaven' or 'Jacob's Ladder'. Serendipitously or synchronistically the building Harvard gave the poets to use as an office had a ladder that went up to the roof.

David was a bit 'flipped out' one day. He had not gotten much sleep and had smoked a little marijuana. At dawn, he walked up the ladder to the top and he looked at the gym and the ivy across the way and he noticed that there was a flock of birds in the ivy. "I believed they were sending me messages. They were passing messages on from other flocks of birds. I realized that they had a global communications network. I was ecstatic. . . . We're talking pure ecstasy."

I asked him what the message was.

"I don't remember specifically. But it had something to do with telling me that what I was doing was okay, was meaningful, was part of a greater plan."

This reminded him as we were talking of an experience he had ten years later as an environmental protection activist. "There was a train carrying hydrogen bombs. They call it the White Train. We blocked it in the northwest three times. I was in front of it all three times. I felt the same sense of purity as when I saw the birds. You know you're in the right place and you're loving and you're feeling connected."

Incarceration and Chemical Torture

Pressures mounted and David continued to be plagued by a sense of insecurity. His behavior was sufficiently eccentric, although not in the least dangerous, that he was committed to McLean's Hospital in Belmont, Massachusetts, against his will. "It's Harvard's teaching hospital. . . . It looks like a country club from the outside but it's all connected by tunnels inside, you seldom see the outside. . . . I was put into the hospital, put into my bedroom, and I sat down and they came in with the

Thorazine. And they said, 'Okay, take this', and I said, 'No, thank you'. I was in there singing to myself and I had a top-of-the-world kind of feeling."

"You really felt good?"

I did. Yes. And they kept pushing the cup of Thorazine toward me. So I poured it on the ground. And for that crime they immediately came in and brought me to solitary confinement and forcibly injected me. Then they made me go back after a day or two in there and mop up the Thorazine on the floor. You know, they took me to solitary, they held me down and pulled down my clothes and gave me the injection. I felt as if I had been raped. I wiped up the Thorazine with my hair to outrage them with my 'submissiveness'.

The drugs caused me all kinds of problems. I couldn't see. I could not read my music or see across the room. I thought my eyes were going bad. The subjective feeling is actually one of disturbance. It's important for people to know that it's not a tranquilizing effect at all. What you feel is a sense of inner turmoil. Viewed from the outside you may look less agitated because you're all mixed up and you're not going to make much noise or show any spirit.

I had difficulty thinking. I remember once trying to make a list of the books I needed from class and not being able to finish the list. I had difficulty moving my tongue which I really resent because I still have residual effects today. I felt like the rats who were given Thorazine in 1950. Thorazine was first tried on rats in December 1950. The French researchers were looking at a range of chemicals trying out different ones, looking to find one that would cause "maximal behavioral disruption". They had a rat trained to climb a rope for food. They finally tried Thorazine—they did not have a name for it yet—but they gave this chemicals to the rat and the rat would go to the rope and would not be able to decide whether to climb the rope for the food. It would panic. It was immobilized. Then they decided, 'This is the one we will use'. They were using it supposedly for other medical purposes . . . but within a year or two it was being given to mental patients. That's one reason why so many people who continue to take these drugs when they get out of the hospital seem to lack the motivation to do things. They will not even climb the rope for the food, metaphorically speaking.

A psychiatrist tried it on herself in the early 1950s and she said she felt as though she was dying, she couldn't get angry at anything. That's how I felt. A few years ago two Israeli psychiatrists took Haldol [a similar neuroleptic drug] and they reported they were unable to work, to think, to even answer a telephone.

David said that forcible druggings were routine and were not restricted to occasions when the 'patient' was agitated or threatened violence. "You see a pattern in all three of my hospitalizations. Any display of spirit was considered to be the enemy and they just looked for that." For example, one time David was attending a 'patient government' meeting. A patient complained that one of the staff members had promised to take him for an ice cream and then defaulted on the promise. David went to find the staff member. He said, "John, Joe would like you to come to the meeting to find out why you did not go for ice cream." John ignored David, who then became angry and said, "Go to the meeting now." John handed David a cookie. David crumbled it in his hand. "Immediately they started to get mental health workers all over the place. I said, 'Wait a minute. Just because I crumbled a cookie? I'll put it in the garbage.' Which I did. But it was too late. It turned into another forced drugging."

David described another demeaning experience he had. "I needed a dime for the pay phone and a nurse came by and I asked her for a dime, which she gave me. And I was trying to be cheerful even though I was on drugs. A psychiatrist was walking by and said, 'Excuse me, what are you going to be giving that nurse in return for the dime?' And I said, 'A smile!' And he said, 'That's the sickest thing I ever heard.' And that hurt me . . . and it helped me to realize their game: either through drugs or words to break you down."

In his senior year David learned about the mental patients' liberation movement that had formed in Cambridge. "I went to Phillips Brooks House, which is a social service agency for Harvard students. I said, 'Look, you should have something about mental patients' rights in here. It's terrible in those places'. One of the women said, 'Let's meet for lunch', which we did and she told me about the Mental Patients' Liberation Front [MPLF] in Cambridge." David joined the organization, went to meetings, gave legal advice to people who called the office, went to demonstrations, and helped to start a drop-in center for former mental patients.

Rebel with a Cause

The mental-health experts told David that he was schizophrenic and needed to stay on medication for the rest of his life. Each time he was released from the hospital he stopped taking the drugs. Harvard required him to take psychiatric drugs to attend. He graduated from Harvard *cum laude* in 1977. He beat the system.

The possibility of making the kind of major life transition represented by Harvard activated David's fears of failure. The working-class boy who made it big, made it to Harvard, and 'flipped out', suddenly found himself facing the worst threat of all: the destruction of all his dreams and reduction to the status of non-person by the mental health establishment.

But he did not capitulate. He was too strong a spirit to be inducted into the role of chronic mental patient. He did exactly what therapists like Jay Haley recommend: as soon as he got out of the hospital he went back to 'normal' life.

I asked David if at any point they had persuaded him he was mentally ill. "I never really, internally, bought the diagnosis. And I never have. My parents would say, 'You know, you really just have to trust somebody'. I was not being supported by the mental health system. I was experiencing new aspects of myself —spiritual, emotional, mystical—but this was happening in a rapid and unassisted way. By help I do not mean someone to stuff it back in, but to help in the process of birth."

David's independence of spirit was a trait he possessed for a long time and helped him to lead others. "I was a rebel with a cause since I was a kid. I published a radical newspaper when I was nine years old, and again at twelve years old, that was censored by my local grade school." In high school he was in the student-empowerment movement and in the anti-Vietnam war movement. In college he remained critical of the 'power system', including Harvard, corporate dominance of America, and authoritarian social relationships.

David's sense of self is defined in broader terms than being a Harvard graduate. "I'm not going to totally reject the accomplishment of getting in there. But I recognized it now as a very narrow aspect of my being. Although of course it is a very unusual thing to graduate in four years with five so-called hospitalizations."

When he finished college, MPLF supplied a great deal of his support. David continued to go to support group meetings and on MPLF wilderness hikes, he became romantically involved with a woman activist in the movement, who helped him improve his nutrition, and he became a vegetarian. He has worked as a volunteer and as a worker for a variety of social causes since 1974. After several years in Boston, supporting himself through office work, David travelled for two years.

In 1982 he helped to organize the International Conference on Human Rights and Against Psychiatric Oppression, which took place in Toronto. After the conference he was excited and had gone without sleep for several days. He began to feel distressed. He was staying in a friend's loft.

> I decided that I would take care of myself. I would lie in bed until I slept. I felt calmer after some sleep. But I was in an altered state. I'd go outside and I'd see construction workers and I'd think these are human beings dressed as construction workers, like actors playing out this experience. Despite this I realized I would be a calm person. I called myself 'The Calm Lithuanian'. I would experience these bizarre thoughts and not panic. And there's a grain of truth here: just because someone is wearing a little plastic cap and has a little sign on their back does not mean that's their identity. I was looking at the person as a whole person and it struck me as funny that they're also playing this little game by digging in the ground and wearing this hat. I have the skill now to experience these things without panicking or getting carried away.

In 1983 David moved to Eugene, Oregon. He continues to edit *Dendron* and to make a salary as an organizer for the movement against nuclear weapons and nuclear power plants. He has been active in the movement to protect the wilderness old-growth areas in Oregon.

> These old-growth wilderness areas are being rampantly cut down. They are Douglas old-growth, Douglas fir, with incredible diversity of species, more living matter per square foot than anywhere on the Earth. The ancient forest evokes feelings very similar to the non-linear states psychiatry is attempting to destroy. Cutting all the old growth down is a violation against nature. I am connected to nature. It's a violation against me. People trying to preserve their natural areas is a very important struggle.

David envisions a global non-violent revolution. He sees people coming together.

> As long as we're alone we can be numbed by the destruction of the planet's ecosystem, by poverty, racism, sexism. We're like deer with the headlights in our eyes. We can't run off the road. But if we organize and support each other our spirits will be lifted so we'll have the strength to fight back."

The mental liberation movement can assist overall societal transformation—a non-violent revolution—in two ways. Two of these are by fighting the tyranny of normality, and teaching the skills of empowering ourselves to lift our own emotions.

With all due respect, I feel a vital part of the human spirit is The Fool. I love this part of ourselves. Our essence of foolishness is a key lesson of the environmental movement: That humans are interrelated with all of nature in such complexity, we should therefore walk as gently and humbly as possible. When a macho business person arrogantly tinkers with nature by, for instance, building a nuclear power plant and ignoring its waste, they deny the foolish essence of their humanity, ironically making themselves more foolish, but also more dangerous. They act as Death Clowns, if you will. How easily their self-interest bends their logic. Unfortunately, their so-called 'delusion' is far more dangerous than those of us actually labeled 'psychotic'.

Today, the unwritten rules which weave our social fabric catalyze a mass adaptation to this Death Clown behavior. The crime of our century has in fact been obedience, not deviance. Those who violate the very core of behavioral fascism, such as many in our movement, can contribute to overthrowing this tyranny of normality.

Our movement also shows people that even a survivor of terrible spirit-destroying economic, social and psychiatric oppression can still overcome. One method we have explored is user-owned mutual support. The idea that individuals can get together as equals and consciously affect—uplift—each other's emotions, lives, and even their biochemistry, is heresy. In fact, that was one reason witches were burned: They formed groups of wise women, linked to the wildness of nature, who through ritual gained power over their own minds and feelings.

The hierarchical, technocratic state we live in has been useful at times. But now it is deadly to Earth itself.

Our movement is part of the transformation by pointing out the unspoken, super-powerful, absurd dictatorship of an enforced sanity. And we can help nurture non-violent revolution by showing everyone has the power to transcend numbness and despair, and keep creative, democratic spirits strong. Through humility and mutual support, humanity can gain the confidence to creatively overcome the dominant world view, hopefully non-violently if at all conceivably possible.

Beating the System

None of the individuals interviewed here was responded to by the system in a therapeutic manner. None of them found places of hospitality operated by mental health professionals. None of them was helped to master the problems causing their distress.

Instead, in the time of their greatest vulnerability they were placed in gulags where their bodies were assaulted and their spirits were violated in the name of 'psychiatric treatment'. The mental health system is a well-oiled machine that destroys the hopes and dreams of millions of vulnerable souls, wreaks havoc on their bodies, and inducts them into becoming chronic mental patients.

The nine survivors who testify in this book (the seven above plus Leonard Frank and George Ebert) refused to allow their soul's fire to be extinguished in exchange for the spurious security offered to them. They refused to accept that they were mentally damaged. They bore witness to the power of the human spirit.

Their testimony dramatically substantiated criticisms of the medical model made over the last 30 years. From the perspective of the mental health establishment, these individuals are chronically mentally ill. From the alternative perspective presented here, these individuals are survivors of psychological and physical attacks on their being by mental-health professionals. They are pioneers who defied the mental health establishment, who refused to capitulate and to accept the role of chronic mental patient that mental-health workers attempted to induct them into. Their story is *not* the story of individuals who 'recovered' from mental illnesses, but of individuals who had the independence of spirit and the breadth of vision to free themselves from the psychological servitude that the mental health establishment attempted to impose upon them 'for their own good'. These are not individuals with defective minds; on the contrary, they are among the most aware, sensitive human beings on the planet.

These individuals beat the system. They got off psychiatric drugs. They went back to work or school. Today they lead 'normal' lives. They have refused to be indoctrinated into believing that they suffer from a chronic disease. They realize that the army of psychologists, psychiatrists, and social workers who rushed to their aid in their times of distress were attempting to undermine their self-confidence. These individuals succeeded in resolving their own life crises in spite of the mental health establishment's attempt to induct them into the role of chronic mental patients. Their experiences bear out the arguments of the critics of institutional psychiatry. The debilitating effects of psychiatric drugs, the absence of genuine therapy, the attempt of numerous authorities to convince them that they never would or could be normal, their difficulty in finding even one therapist among thousands who would regard them as individuals rather than as specimens of chronic mental pathology—all of this has been attested to by the survivors interviewed above. Each of these individuals is keenly aware that he or she narrowly escaped the fate of becoming a chronic mental patient and being herded into day-treatment centers, being maintained on debilitating psychiatric drugs, and being consigned to the demeaning status of 'the chronically mentally ill'. All of them are now leading creative, challenging lives with no signs of 'psychopathology'—except, of course, to the mental-health worker who is trained to see pathology everywhere. That is not to say, of course, that their lives are free of problems and difficulties. As Thomas Szasz wrote,

> The concept of mental illness . . . serves mainly to obscure the everyday fact that life for most people is a continuous struggle, not for biological survival, but for a 'place in the sun', 'peace of mind', or some other value. . . .
>
> The myth of mental illness encourages us to believe in its logical corollary: that social intercourse would be harmonious, satisfying, and the secure basis of a good life were it not for the disrupting influences of mental illness or psychopathology. However, universal human happiness, in this form at least, is but another example of wishful fantasy. I believe that human happiness, or well-being, is possible—not just for a select few, but on a scale hitherto unimaginable. But this can be achieved only if many men, not just a few, are willing and able to confront frankly, and tackle courageously, their ethical, personal, and social conflicts.[1]

[1]Thomas Szasz, *Primary Values and Major Contentions* (New York: Prometheus, 1983), 66

Psychiatry has historically perpetrated all kinds of assaults on individuals in the name of protecting them from mental illness. And then the consequences of these assaults are attributed to the ravages of mental illness. How can we advance the cause of human liberation when those who now have the power—the mental health experts and their allies—are so emotionally and financially invested in the massive consensually-validated delusional system that they have constructed, that they are unwilling to listen to the word of truth? The cogs grind on, the wheels turn and the mental health machine races toward the abyss as if to its own salvation.

Carl Jung said, "Learn your theories well but put them aside when you confront the mystery of the living soul." There is no room in the mental health system for the recognition of the mystery of the living soul. There are no interstices in institutional mental health where such a sacramental meeting could take place.

The individuals whose stories I have recounted triumphed because they all reached the point where they began to question the authority of the secular priesthood that informed them they were irreparably damaged and doomed. As George Ebert told me once, "If I had accepted what they told me about myself I couldn't accept myself." Kristin openly defied the experts. "You're manic-depressive," they said. "I've never been manic." "Well, you're depressed then." "No, I'm not depressed, I'm sad." She remarked to me, "It was natural for me to be sad. My marriage had failed, my parents sucked rocks, I have nowhere to go except back to the fiancé I was fighting because of my parents. What was I supposed to be so thrilled about?"

Certainly the human soul will face obstacles in its life journey, and may become dispirited or discouraged. This does not justify the conclusion that the psyche is 'damaged' or 'flawed'. This assertion is not made on the basis of objective biological grounds. Nor is it a statement about 'biology': 'You have deeply-rooted psychopathology'. 'You have a biochemical imbalance'. 'You are genetically defective'. These are metaphors that imply the person is inferior, lacking in worth. The basis for making this ascription is that the individual does not conform to the Priesthood's arbitrary cultural criteria of normality. If Jesus Christ were to return today he would no doubt be considered mentally defective by the mental health experts, as would Elijah, Elisha, Isaiah, or Jeremiah.

The good news is that a process of spiritual transformation has begun on this planet. Almost all of the subjects interviewed had a glimpse of another reality, a higher power, a vision of the interconnectedness of all beings. They honored these visions.

The veil of ignorance that envelops our species is so dense that we fail to realize that outside our artificial cocoon there is a universe that is suffused with sunlight and color. So often we fail to notice what is unfamiliar, what is strange. We do not notice the jewels that glisten in the darkness of our ignorance, since we tell ourselves that these are apparitions, and apparitions are madness, and madness must be banished at any cost!

"Something is happening here but you don't know what it is, do you, Mr. Jones?" sang Bob Dylan. The process of spiritual awakening has begun. All of the individuals interviewed in this book are witness to that fact. We do not know where it is leading but those of us who have awakened know that it must not, it cannot, it will not be aborted by those who seek to perpetuate the *status quo* at all costs.

"The crime of our century has in fact been obedience, not deviance," David said. The experts who told the heroes in this book, 'You are a schizophrenic' and 'You must take these drugs for the rest of your life" were only following orders; only doing what they were schooled to do. Now is the time to revolt. Now is the time to build a movement against the mental health establishment. This will help to create the space for bringing a new social and cultural order into existence.

PART TWO

Heretics, Apostates, and Infidels

*To follow after the highest in us
may seem to be to live
dangerously . . . but by that
danger comes victory and
security. To rest in or follow
after an inferior potentiality
may seem safe, rational,
comfortable, easy, but it ends
badly, in some futility or in a
mere circling, down the abyss
or in a stagnant morass. Our
right and natural road is
towards the summits.*

—SRI AUROBINDO
*THE REALIZATION OF THE IDEAL
OF HUMAN UNITY*

Critics of the Concept of Mental Illness

In 1961, Thomas Szasz published *The Myth of Mental Illness.* In that book, Szasz argued that the concept of 'mental illness' is a metaphor, and that as a metaphor it does not illuminate the experience or behavior of the individual to whom it is applied, but on the contrary it obscures essential features of the individual's behavior and of the human situation in general. Szasz argued that the term was used to stigmatize deviants from social norms and to deprive them of their democratic rights and responsibilities.

Since Szasz's work first appeared, numerous books and essays have been published attacking the premises of what has come to be termed 'the medical model' of human psychology. I believe that these critical works demonstrate that the medical model in psychology lacks any kind of scientific or humanistic justification.

There are a number of variations of the medical model. All are based on the same simple formula. The two medical models that dominate in the field today are the psychoanalytic model and the biochemical imbalance model; the former is rapidly losing ground to the latter. Most mental-health workers accept an amalgam of the two. Thomas Scheff succinctly describes the psychoanalytic-medical version: "The basic model upon which psychoanalysis is constructed is the disease model, in that it portrays neurotic behavior as unfolding relentlessly out of a defective psychological system contained within the body."[1] In the case of the biochemical model, one would say that it portrays neurotic or 'sick' behavior as unfolding relentlessly out of a defective *metabolic* or *physiological* system contained within the body. In the psychoanalytic model, the psychological system is ostensibly defective as a result primarily of traumas suffered by the individual in the first several years of his life, when he or she is said to be most impressionable. In the case of the biochemical

---

[1]Thomas Scheff, *Being Mentally Ill* (Chicago: Aldine, 1966), 9

imbalance model, the defective system is a result of inexplicable genetic goofs. The basic algorithm or formula of the medical model is simple: sick behavior issues relentlessly from a defective system within the individual. It is simple but problematic.

In the first place, the judgment that particular behavior is 'sick' is based on criteria that are culturally determined and questionable. The controversial nature of these judgments is disguised by using medical terms to describe behavior that the mental health establishment does not approve of. This fact has been recognized by both Szasz and Laing among others. Tuberculosis and pneumonia, for example, are names for processes that are judged to be pathological on biological grounds: they clearly threaten to shorten or impair the life of the organism. Consequently, there is little controversy, within the field of medicine, about the fundamental concept of disease: one does not find a group of dissenters claiming that it is unfair to describe a person who is manifesting the symptoms of pneumonia as ill. Furthermore, to say that a person is physically ill is not to say that his or her mind, psyche or soul is impaired, which is a much more incriminating assertion.

But in the case of what is defined as neurosis, or psychosis, or mental illness, the dominant cultural values influence what the experts define as pathological. But are these cultural values to be accepted as absolutes? And is not the use of the term 'mental illness' a devious strategy to undermine the self-respect of those who deviate from the status quo? In the nineteenth century, masturbation was considered to be symptomatic of a disease. Homosexuality was considered a disease until 1973, when thanks to lobbying by homosexual psychiatrists within the American Psychiatric Association it was decided by a rather close vote that it was no longer a disease (as long as the homosexual likes it; homosexuality continues to be classed as a disease when the homosexual dislikes being homosexual). Internists do not vote at conventions to decide whether one should classify tuberculosis as a disease. For this reason, it's difficult to refute Szasz's and Laing's argument that the term 'mental illness' is used to stigmatize individuals who deviate from social norms. This suggests, of course, that therapists may be creating problems for individuals rather than helping to alleviate them.

Anthropology adds additional weight to the argument against the medical model. In 1934, Ruth Benedict, one of the founders of anthropology, wrote, "It is clear the culture may value and make socially available even highly unstable human types. If it chooses to treat their peculiarities as the most valued variants in human behavior, the individuals in question will rise to the occasion and perform their social roles without reference to the ideas of the usual types who can make social adjustments and those who cannot. Those who function inadequately in any society are not those with certain fixed 'abnormal' traits, but may well be those whose responses have received no support in the institutions of their culture. The weakness of these aberrants is in great measure illusory. It springs not from the fact that they are lacking in necessary vigor, but that they are individuals whose native responses are not reaffirmed by society. They are, as Sapir phrases it, 'alienated from an impossible world'."[2]

Over 30 years later, R.D. Laing argued that indeed the person who was most likely to be labelled severely mentally ill was saner than those who were doing the labeling, that he was "alienated from an impossible world", as Ruth Benedict put it. In Laing's words, "Our society may itself have become biologically dysfunctional, and some forms of schizophrenic alienation from the alienation of society may have a socio-biological function that we have not recognized."[3]

Two aspects of Laing's argument should be noted. In the first place, he was one of the first to redirect attention to the social context in which behavior labelled 'pathological' took place. By doing this he was able to demonstrate the intelligibility of behavior which, abstracted from its social context, seems unintelligible and thus is likely to be labeled pathological by individuals ignoring its context. Laing was influenced here by the work of Bateson, Jackson, Haley, and Weakland,[4] all of whom except Bateson later became family therapists and who did the classic study of schizophrenics and their families which showed that, as Laing put it, "*No* schizophrenic has been studied whose disturbed pattern of communication has not been shown to be a reflection of, and reaction to, the disturbed and disturbing pattern characterizing his or her family of origin."[5] In other words, puzzling or dysfunctional behavior does not unfold

[2]Ruth Benedict, *Patterns of Culture* (New York: Houghton-Mifflin, 1934), 270

[3]R.D. Laing, *The Politics of Experience* (New York: Pantheon, 1968), 120

[4]G. Bateson, D. O. Jackson, J. Haley, and J. Weakland, 'Towards a Theory of Schizophrenia', *Behavioral Science,* Volume 1, November 25th, 1956

[5]Laing, *The Politics of Experience, op cit,* 114

relentlessly out of a defective system within the body. The metaphor of mental illness obscures this fundamental fact.

Secondly, Laing claimed that psychiatrically labelled people were in fact more aware, more sensitive, more spiritually inclined, and thus likely to be discriminated against by a materialistically oriented establishment. Laing's meditation on schizophrenia in his classic book, *The Politics of Experience,* was an attack on the spiritual vacuity of modern civilization.

This claim is actually lent credence by Julian Silverman's seminal article, 'Shamans and Acute Schizophrenia', published in *The American Anthropologist* in 1967. Reviewing a broad range of anthropologic material, Silverman compared the initiatory ordeal typically experienced by the novice shaman to what psychiatrists term a schizophrenic episode; he is not referring to the experiences of the veteran shaman but to the initiand. Silverman concludes, "Significant differences between acute schizophrenics and shamans are not found in the sequence of underlying psychological events that define their abnormal experiences."[6] The major difference Silverman did find was that in primitive society these abnormal experiences were valued and individuals were provided with an interpretive framework that enabled them to make sense of these experiences and to integrate them into their daily lives. This was part of the process of being initiated into the vocation of the shaman. Silverman termed shamanism a "unique resolution of a basic life crisis". In the modern world, these experiences are not valued but "invalidated", as Laing had argued, and the elders of this society do not present the individual in crisis with the option of shamanism— or anything other than chronic mental patienthood—as a means of resolving his or her suffering.

In a paper that I delivered several years ago to a conference of ex-'mental patients', I wrote, "The implications of this are staggering. Yesterday's shaman is today's chronic schizophrenic! The kind of person who, in a bygone era, would have been initiated into the vocation of shaman, medicine man, spiritual healer, is now likely to be initiated into the role of tragic-victim-of-the-most-serious-mental-illness-known-to-modern-civilization."[7]

[6]Julian Silverman, 'Shamans and Acute Schizophrenia', *American Anthropologist,* 69, 1967, 21

[7]Seth Farber, 'The Challenge of Cosmic Optimism', *Inside Out Magazine,* Vol 1., No. 2, November-December 1988, 12

Mircea Eliade, the prominent historian of religion, wrote that the shaman "has succeeded in integrating into consciousness a considerable number of experiences that, for the profane world, are reserved for dreams, madness or post-mortem states. The shamans and mystics of primitive society are considered—and rightly—to be superior beings; their magico-religious powers also find expression in an extension of their mental capacities. The shaman is the man who knows and remembers, that is, who understands the mysteries of life and death. . . ."[8]

Silverman's article and Eliade's studies, both of shamanism and puberty initiation rites in pre-modern cultures, lend weight to another one of Laing's contentions: that the 'schizophrenic breakdown', when left to run its natural course, constitutes a natural process of spiritual death and regeneration. The crisis that precedes regeneration is frequently a total crisis leading to the 'disintegration of the personality', as Eliade describes a shamanic crisis. "In no rite or myth do we find the initiatory death as something final, but always as the *condition sine qua non* of a transition to another mode of being, a trial indispensable to regeneration; that is, to the beginning of a new life."[9] The procedures of the mental health establishment abort a process whose ultimate aim is spiritual rebirth, the creation of a new being, the formation of a more mature sense of personal identity.

Sarbin corroborated this point in 'Self-Reconstitutive Processes'. He demonstrated that a death-rebirth process takes place in contexts as diverse as Alcoholics Anonymous, Christian monastic mysticism, religious conversions, shamanic initiations, brainwashing and in successful psychotherapy.[10] We have also seen that this same process took place in the survivors whose stories were told above.

The idea that individuals until recently labelled schizophrenic (now precisely the same kinds of individuals are more likely to be labelled 'manic-depressive') were somehow more spiritually inclined, in other words, possessed particular qualities that might be looked at as gifts in another context, was ridiculed by the Establishment. The idea that 'schizophrenia' was potentially regenerative was ignored. Article after article denounced Laing

[8]Mircea Eliade, *Birth and Rebirth* (New York: Harper, 1958), 102

[9]Mircea Eliade, *Myths, Dreams, and Mysteries* (New York: Harper and Row, 1975), 224

[10]T. Sarbin and N. Adler, 'Self-Reconstitutive Processes', *Psychoanalytic Review*, 1971, 56(4), 599–616

as an unrealistic romanticist who was impervious to the tremendous suffering of the 'mentally ill'.

The establishment turned a blind eye to the cogent arguments made by Laing and others that it was in fact their own very practices that greatly exacerbated and perpetuated the suffering of 'the mentally ill'. They failed to acknowledge that terms such as 'mental illness', 'damaged ego', 'deeply rooted pathology' or, more recently, 'biochemical imbalance' were merely metaphors. Other metaphors, equally or more fitting, and less degrading, could be substituted, as Sarbin and Mancuso argued. These terms are metaphors insofar as they refer not to an actual corporeal body, but to the person's incorporeal mind or psyche, which is the Greek word for soul, the core of the person's being. The ascription of such metaphors is in fact the first step in a process of degradation.

> If the label of disrespect is applied by an individual or a group empowered to apply such labels, the society goes to work to treat the individual as a non-person . . . The pejorative labels provide a means of codifying the answers to the *who are you* question, and to designate a *degraded social identity.* The pejorative label, for example, schizophrenic, is assigned by mental health workers. The label serves the same function as visible stigmata of degradation. . . . The stigmata of degradation serve the purpose of identifying non-persons. [Sarbin and Mancuso use the term 'non-persons' to describe individuals who have been deprived of all social status and of the right and privilege of being held responsible for their actions.] Even branding has been used to designate such declared non-persons as harlots, heretics, and slaves. In modern times, non-visible stigmata in the form of diagnostic labels have been employed —mental patients, psychotics, schizophrenics, lunatics, etc.[11]

A variety of sociologists and psychologists began to look at the psychological and physical processes that individuals were subjected to once they were defined as 'mentally ill'. Szasz had argued that this particular definition was a pretext for depriving individuals of their democratic rights: "How are involuntary psychiatric interventions—and the many other medical violations of individual freedom—justified or made possible? By calling people *patients,* imprisonment *hospitalization,* and torture *therapy;* and by calling uncomplaining individuals *sufferers,*

---

[11]Theodore Sarbin and James Mancuso, *Schizophrenia: Medical Diagnosis or Moral Verdict?* (New York: Pergamon, 1980), 217

medical and mental health personnel who infringe on their liberty and dignity *therapists,* and the things the latter do to the former *treatments.* That is why such terms as *mental health* and the *right to treatment* now so effectively conceal that psychiatry is involuntary servitude."[12]

The sociologist Erving Goffman examined the 'scientific' and 'medical' procedures that typically take place in mental hospitals, and showed that they were not scientific procedures at all, that they were "rituals of degradation" (he borrowed that phrase from the sociologist Garfinkle).

> Mental hospitals bureaucratically institutionalize this extremely wide mandate [to pronounce the final verdict on the individual's past] by formally basing their treatment of the patient on his diagnosis and hence upon the psychiatric view of his past. . . . The case record is an important expression of this mandate. The dossier is apparently not regularly used, however, to record occasions when the patient showed capacity to cope honorably and effectively with difficult life situations. Nor is the case record typically used to provide a rough average or sampling of his past conduct. One of its purposes is to show the way in which the patient is 'sick' and the reasons why it was right to commit him and is right currently to keep him committed; and this is done by extracting from his whole life course a list of those incidents that have or might have had 'symptomatic' significance. The misadventures of his parents or siblings that might suggest a 'taint' may be cited. Early acts in which the patient appeared to have shown bad judgment or emotional disturbances will be recorded. Occasions when he acted in a way which the layman would consider immature, sexually perverted, weak-willed, childish, ill-considered, impulsive and crazy may be described. . . . In addition, the record will describe the state on arrival at the hospital—and this is not likely to be a time of tranquility and ease for him.[13]

In other words, the so-called neutral diagnosis is not a balanced picture, but is based on a selective focus on those incidents in the individual's life where he or she has failed to cope or has acted inappropriately. His or her successes are ignored. The case record, of course, is the basis upon which a 'diagnosis' and a 'prognosis' will be based. The individual and

---

[12]Thomas Szasz, *The Theology of Medicine* (New York: Harper and Row, 1977), xix

[13]Erving Goffman, *Asylums* (New York: Doubleday, 1961), 155–56

his or her family will be told that it has been determined scientifically that he or she suffers from a 'chronic mental illness' and that he or she must drastically lower his or her expectations about what he or she can accomplish in life.

Rosenhan's 'On Being Sane in Insane Places', published in 1973, was only the most dramatic of a number of studies demonstrating that there is in fact nothing scientific about psychiatric diagnosis. The psychiatrist or other mental worker has a tendency to see 'pathology' everywhere. Furthermore, the study demonstrates that the labelling process is irreversible: once a person is labelled schizophrenic, there is virtually no way he or she can get rid of the label. In Rosenhan's study, 'normal' people, that is to say, individuals who worked as professionals (teachers, lawyers, psychologists, and so forth) and who had no previous history of psychiatric hospitalization, pretended they were hearing sounds in order to be admitted into psychiatric wards; once in the wards they acted as they normally would. *Not a single one* of the staff of psychiatrists, psychologists, social workers, or aides suspected that these were in fact 'normal' people. Rosenhan wrote that, "having once been labelled schizophrenic there is nothing the pseudo-patient can do to overcome the tag. The tag profoundly colors others' perception of him and his behavior."[14] Indeed, Rosenhan found from an examination of the staff notes and case reports that the patients' behavior and past history were interpreted in such a way as to confirm the diagnosis of 'schizophrenia'.[15] "Many of the pseudo-patients' normal behaviors were overlooked entirely or profoundly misinterpreted to make them fit into the assumed reality."[16] When the patients were finally discharged, they were discharged with the diagnosis, "schizophrenia in remission".[17] In other words, all of these individuals were told that they were chronically mentally ill and were in perpetual danger of going crazy again. Although Rosenhan's article caused a controversy in the intellectual world, it had no impact on any of the practices and procedures in mental hospitals or in outpatient clinics.

All of these investigations and critiques demonstrated a sensitivity to environmental variables and to the *context* in

---

[14]D. Rosenhan, 'On Being Sane in Insane Places', in Paul Watzlawick (ed.), *The Invented Reality* (New York: Norton, 1984), 125

[15]*Ibid.*, 125–130

[16]*Ibid.*, 125

[17]*Ibid.*, 122

which behavior takes place that is completely lacking in the adherents to the medical model. It now began to appear that much of the distress or dysfunctional behavior did *not* proceed relentlessly out of a defective psychological system or a defective physiological system, as Scheff had put it.

The family therapy movement, which began to develop in the 1950s, provided a new perspective from which to view 'deviant' behavior.[18] The innovators in this field rejected the idea of mental illness. Behavior that appeared to be crazy or pathological was in actuality a response to unacknowledged and unnegotiated conflicts within the family. These conflicts ultimately evoked the fear of a splintering of the family, such as separation or divorce. Alternatively, even in the absence of potentially divisive conflicts, 'symptomatic behavior' might appear at the time of an impending transition to a new phase in the individual or family life cycle, which inevitably raises the spectre of disintegration. Leaving home, getting married, having children mark transitions that might potentially lead one member of the family to act sympomatically, in order to keep the family together, to restore stability at any price. Haley wrote, "The symptom is a signal that a family has difficulty in getting past a stage in the life cycle."[19] The task of the therapist is to facilitate these transitions.

The symptomatic behavior did not unfold relentlessly out of a defective system within the individual. Three points are relevant here. Firstly, the 'identified patient'—this was a phrase family therapists invented to express their critical stance toward the idea of mental illness—was expressing anxiety experienced by other family members as well. Secondly, the symptomatic behavior was viewed by family therapists as an indication not that there was something wrong with the psychological or physiological system of the individual, but rather that the family as a whole was relating in a dysfunctional manner. Thirdly, the symptomatic behavior was not the *result* of a pathological process, but was a goal-directed act (however unconscious or barely conscious). It was the identified patient's solution to the threat or imagined threat of the disintegration of the

[18]Lynn Hoffman, *Foundations of Family Therapy* (New York: Basic Books, 1981). Jay Haley, *Problem-Solving Therapy* (New York: Harper and Row, 1976)

[19]Jay Haley, *Uncommon Therapy; The Psychiatric Techniques of Milton H. Erickson* (New York: Norton, 1973), 42

family; it was a solution that maintained unity while warding off the threat of change.

Traditional therapy can be destructive for a number of reasons. In the first place, it confirms the identified patient's status as a mentally ill person: thus, unity is achieved at the cost of the autonomy of the individual defined as an identified patient. Family conflicts continue to be unacknowledged and everybody joins together in order to sympathize with and help the poor 'chronically mentally ill patient'. Secondly, of course, no therapy takes place insofar as the underlying family problems remain untouched. The symptomatic behavior is now sanctioned by the Mental Health Establishment, which acts as if this behavior is beyond the control of the individual. This was a powerful critique of the traditional medical model—and it worked.

Pioneers in the family therapy movement such as Minuchin,[20] Haley[21] and Watzlawick[22] were explicitly and implicitly critical of psychoanalytic theory which postulated that the individual was 'damaged' because of events in early childhood. From the family therapy perspective, the causes of the individual's dysfunctional behavior were irrelevant. Unlike the Freudians, the family therapists did not believe that the individual was pursuing irrational or illusory goals, such as trying to obtain Mommy's approval through the medium of another adult. On the contrary, their observations and interventions were consistent with the thesis that their clients were motivated by the desire to create fulfilling relationships in the present. The problem was rather that the clients had developed patterns of behavior that subverted their ability to achieve these goals. Theoretical discussions of the intricacy of the psyche provided a socially acceptable means of intellectual stimulation for mental-health professionals, and it maintained their social status as intrepid explorers of the netherworld of the mind. Unfortunately, it bypassed the more mundane task of helping their clients to achieve the goals for which they sought help in the first place.

Furthermore, the psychoanalytic dogma that individuals are programmed in the first few years of their lives and will continue to re-enact those programs again and again unless they spent years in psychotherapy did not stand up to empirical scrutiny.

---

[20] Salvador Minuchin, *Families and Family Therapy* (Cambridge: Harvard University Press, 1974)

[21] Jay Haley, *Leaving Home* (New York: McGraw Hill, 1980)

[22] Paul Watzlawick et al., *Change: Principles of Problem Formation and Problem Resolution* (New York: Norton, 1974)

Kenneth Gergen (1977)[23] has termed this view "the stability orientation" and points out that its quintessential feature is its premise that behavior patterns remain stable over time and that the individual is basically predictable. Both Gergen and Jerome Kagan[24] refute the psychoanalytic dogma on the overwhelming preponderance of early childhood experience for later development. The major variable the neo-psychoanalysts stress is anxiety over 'object loss' in the first few years of life. Yet Kagan (1970) noted, "The variation in degree of anxiety over loss of access to attachment figures during the first three years of life predicted no significant behavior in adolescence or adulthood."[25] Although the work of Kagan and Gergen and others supports a more optimistic interpretation of the effect of early childhood experience on later development, there has been no modification of psychoanalytic theory or practice. Nor has this research had much impact on contemporary culture, which Gergen observes has "almost fully accepted the assumption that early experience is vital in shaping adult behavior."[26]

Furthermore, Gergen summarizes the data collected by life-span development researchers which indicate that development is idiosyncratic and unpredictable: "The individual seems fundamentally flexible in most aspects of personal functioning. Significant change in the life course may occur at any time. . . . An immense panoply of developmental forms seems possible; which particular form emerges may depend on a confluence of particulars, the existence of which is fundamentally unsystematic."[27]

If development is idiosyncratic, then psychoanalysts have no justification for placing individuals within 'diagnostic' categories (based on their ostensible degree of mental pathology) and acting as if those categories reflect ontological features of the universe. They have no justification for making predictions about individ-

---

[23]Gergen, 'Stability, Change and Chance in Understanding Human Development. In N. Datan and H. Reese (eds.), *Life Span Developmental Psychology: Dialectical Perspectives* (135–158). New York: Academic Press, 1977

[24]J. Kagan, 'Perspectives on continuity.' In O. Brim and J. Kagan (eds.), *Constancy and Change in Human Development* (26–74). Cambridge: Harvard University Press, 1970

[25]*Ibid.*

[26]Gergen, *op. cit.*, 142

[27]K. Gergen, 'The Emerging Crisis in Life-span Development Theory. In P. Baltes and O. Brim (eds.), *Life-span Development and Behavior* (31–63). New York: Academic Press, 1980, 43

uals' future development—these very predictions themselves constrain individuals' possibilities for change and action as self-fulfilling prophecies. If development depends upon 'unsystematic' factors, then conceivably a problem that seems to be very serious and intractable—for instance, a 'psychotic' breakdown—could resolve itself in the twinkling of an eye. Falling in love could conceivably completely alter the trajectory of a person's previous development.

In 1980, Theodore Sarbin and James Mancuso published their monumental work, *Schizophrenia: Medical Diagnosis or Moral Verdict?* Both authors were professors of psychology and Sarbin in particular was known in social psychology for his numerous contributions over many years to the development of role theory. This book is the most thorough examination and critique of the medical model in psychology. As the Michelson-Morley experiment spelled the end of traditional physics and paved the way for Einstein's theory, so ought Sarbin and Mancuso's work to have put an end to the disease model and paved the way for the kinds of alternative conceptualizations outlined in this book and elsewhere. It is a sad reflection on the mental health professions that by 1988 this book was already out of print. Sarbin and Mancuso meticulously examine in this book 20 years of research, published in the standard psychiatric and psychological journals, designed to prove that schizophrenia is a disease. As Krasner said in the introduction to the book, "Sarbin and Mancuso play fairly in that the 'schizophrenia' research is analyzed within the context of the rules of the scientific game. They demonstrate unequivocally that the research is deficient. To demonstrate with detailed scholarship and research sensitivity in the field of 'schizophrenia' that 'the Emperor has no clothes' is indeed a major accomplishment. . . . The full implications and consequences of the Sarbin-Mancuso alternative conceptualization should, could, and must be developed by the current generation of scientists, practitioners, and students."[28]

Sarbin and Mancuso write after surveying 60 years of research, and carefully scrutinizing the last 20 years, "Not one dependent measure has been identified that would allow a professional diagnostician to make a reliable diagnosis. If schizophrenia could be diagnosed like pneumonia, then 60 years of research would have identified at least one causal agent."[29]

[28]Sarbin and Mancuso, *op. cit.,* xxi
[29]*Ibid.*

Although the researchers in the journals invariably draw the conclusion that schizophrenia is a disease that destroys cognitive and perceptual abilities, the data indicate otherwise. In each experiment, the data reveal only small differences in group means between the performance of schizophrenics and the performance of the control groups on the experimental tasks. This means, as Sarbin and Mancuso note, that the majority of individuals labelled schizophrenics were performing comparably to the majority of people labelled normal. The small differences in the group means indicate that only some of the experimental group were performing less adequately. Sarbin and Mancuso easily account for this difference by examining a number of "disguised variables", such as the effects of psychotropic drugs on the performance of the experimental task.

They conclude that the resolution of a life crisis is forestalled by the mental health workers who initiate a process of transvaluing and degrading individuals' social identity. Their model takes into account what happens to the individual in the context of a mental hospital, where he or she is subjected to the variety of degradation rituals previously mentioned, and isolated and sequestered with other labeled deviants, and denied opportunities to engage in the kind of 'role enactments' that are capable of earning one esteem within the existing social order.

Sarbin and Mancuso's analysis here interfaces with that done by Jay Haley in his book, published in the same year, *Leaving Home,* although neither of them shows any awareness of the other's work. The crisis that an individual faces can only be resolved by extricating him or her from the patient role as quickly as possible and introducing him back into a natural environment where he or she would have the opportunity to engage in the kinds of role-enactments that typically earn one esteem. The mental health establishment *discourages* this process and tells individuals that they have a disease that will prevent them from leading a normal life and engaging in esteem-earning activities.

As Sarbin and Mancuso were fading into obscurity, Peter Breggin launched a new attack with his book, *Psychiatric Drugs: Hazards to the Brain.*[30] Breggin debunked the myth that psychiatric drugs were medications designed to cure specific mental diseases. He showed that the most widely prescribed psychiatric

---

[30]Peter Breggin, *Psychiatric Drugs: Hazards to the Brain* (New York: Springer, 1983)

drugs, the phenothiazines, were in fact drugs that did not have a specific effect on individuals with specific disorders, but had the same general effect on any individual who took such drugs. They are neurotoxic drugs that interfere with higher cortical level functioning and that in general induce a state of "psychic indifference".

The initial promoters of the drugs were quite blunt about the drugs' effects: they produced a "chemical lobotomy" and made it more easy to control the schizophrenic patient. The discoverer of chlorpromazine wrote, "Patients receiving the drug become lethargic. Manic patients often will not object to rest and patients who present management problems become tractable. . . . The patients under treatment display a lack of spontaneous interest in the environment. . . . They tend to remain silent and immobile when left alone and to reply to questions in a slow monotone. . . ."[31] Furthermore, he acknowledges, "Many patients dislike the 'empty' feeling resulting from the reduction of drive and spontaneity which is apparently one of the most characteristic effects of this substance."[32] Revealingly enough, he compares the effects of this drug to a lobotomy. "In the management of pain and terminal cancer cases, chlorpromazine may prove to be a pharmacological substitute for lobotomy."[33]

Laing had written in *The Politics of Experience* that "the condition of alienation, of being asleep, of being unconscious, of being out of one's mind is a condition of normal man."[34] It is not surprising that psychiatrists are quite enthusiastic about a drug that turns restless and discontented individuals into individuals who, like themselves, have made their peace with the *status quo*. As Noyes and Kolb wrote in the 1958 edition of *Modern Clinical Psychiatry*, "If the patient responds well to the drug, he develops an attitude of *indifference*, both to his surroundings and to his symptoms. He shows decreased interest in and response to his hallucinatory experiences and a less assertive expression of his delusional ideas. Even though not somnolent, the patient may lie quietly in bed, unoccupied and staring ahead. He may answer questions readily and to the point but offer little or no spontaneous conversation; however, questioning shows that he is fully aware of his circumstances."[35] In the 1977 edition

---

[31]*Ibid.,* 14

[32]*Ibid.,* 15

[33]*Ibid.,* 15

[34]Laing, *The Politics of Experience, op. cit.*

[35]Peter Breggin, *Psychiatric Drugs: Hazards to the Brain, op. cit.*

of the same book, Kolb repeated: "If the patient responds well to the drug, he develops an attitude of indifference, both to his surroundings and to his symptoms."[36] (The argument that the use of these drugs accounts for the release of many patients from state mental hospitals is questioned in Appendix 2.)

Breggin's argument that these drugs cause serious neurological damage when used for more than a brief period of time is no longer even controversial. This has become so evident that even mainstream psychiatrists cannot deny it. Massive reliance on these drugs has caused an epidemic of tardive dyskinesia. The American Psychiatric Association Task Force report –18 estimated that 60–65 percent of the individuals who take these drugs regularly develop tardive dyskinesia.[37]

Psychiatrists are increasingly relying on Lithium as the drug of choice. This drug also has deleterious effects on the body and brain when used for more than a brief period of time. Its destructive effects are less noticeable, since it does not cause uncontrollable muscular spasms and twitching. Like the phenothiazines, it also produces a feeling of 'psychic indifference'. One of the promoters of this drug described patients who were taking the drug: "It was as if their 'intensity of living' dial had been turned down a few notches. Things do not seem so very important or imperative; there is a greater acceptance of everyday life as it is rather than as one might want it to be; and their spouses report a much more peaceful existence."[38]

Breggin also devoted a book to documenting the destructive consequences of what is euphemistically termed 'electro-shock therapy'.[39] This is a more controversial treatment and its promoters have gone to great lengths to convince the public that the 'new, modified' ECT is in fact a useful therapeutic tool that causes no ill-effects. In the last few years ECT has been increasingly relied upon by psychiatrists and it was estimated in 1978 that 100,000 to 200,000 individuals per year received ECT.[40] (Vigorous promotion of ECT in the last five years leads me to surmise that its use has increased.)

[36]*Ibid.,* 17

[37]*American Psychiatric Task Force,* Report No. 18 (Washington, DC: American Psychiatric Association, 1980)

[38]Breggin, *Psychiatric Drugs: Hazards to the Brain, op. cit.,* 198

[39]Peter Breggin, *Electroshock: Its Brain-Disabling Effects* (New York: Springer, 1979)

[40]*American Psychiatric Task Force,* Report No. 14 (Washington, DC: American Psychiatric Association, 1978)

It's no wonder that so many individuals remain trapped within the mental health system. The brainwashing procedures used to convince them that they are chronically mentally ill are as potent as any of the procedures used in Chinese prisoner-of-war camps. The conditions at mental hospitals, despite the illusion of progress and humanitarian reform, have not changed much since the last century. In 1830, John Connolly, then professor of medicine at the new University College, London, and later to become one of the most famous figures in nineteenth-century English psychiatry, wrote that for two-thirds of the inmates, "confinement is the very reverse of beneficial. It fixes and renders permanent what might have passed away. . . . I have seen numerous examples . . . in which it was evident that . . . a continued residence in the asylum was gradually ruining body and mind. . . . The sanest among us would find it difficult to resist the horrible influences of the place. . . . Patients are subjected . . . to the very circumstances most likely to confuse or destroy the rational and healthy mind."[41]

Criticisms of the medical model have had no effect on public policy. This is perhaps not surprising because of the power of those groups with a vested interest in the perpetuation of the *status quo*. As Krasner noted in his introduction to Sarbin and Mancuso's book, "It would be an interesting exercise in economics and occupational sociology to show in detail how 'schizophrenia' as a disease metaphor has spawned thousands of jobs, not only for the psychiatric team (psychiatrists, clinical psychologists, and social workers), and other mental hospital employees, but also for the pharmaceutical, publishing, hospital supply, and related industries. The first task of any industry is to perpetuate itself and then to expand."[42]

Probably, a good deal less than one percent of the practicing therapists actually believe that 'schizophrenia' or 'manic-depression' do *not* refer to actual diseases but are merely labels applied by one group of human beings to another. Mainstream psychologists' and psychiatrists' response to their critics is to insist that they are, at best, well-meaning but misguided romanticists who fail to understand the plight of the chronically mentally ill. The media merely repeat the official party line on mental illness, and intellectuals in related disciplines have turned a deaf ear to the

[41]Andrew Scull, *Social Order/Mental Disorder* (Berkelely: University of California Press, 1989), 45–46

[42]Sarbin and Mancuso, *op. cit.,* x

critics of the mental health establishment and have been content either to reiterate the Freudian homilies as if they were the word of God or to give their adherence to the doctrine of the genetic defect.

Psychotherapists have ignored the data on experimenter bias which have revolutionary implications. This research shows that we are responsible for the creation and perpetuation of the behaviors that we classify as mental illnesses. Reviewing the literature on this topic, Jerome Frank writes: "To recapitulate the chief findings, an experimenter's expectations can strongly bias the performance of his subject by means of cues so subtle that neither experimenter nor subject need be aware of them." Furthermore, "a therapist cannot avoid biasing his patient's performance in accordance with his own expectations, based on his evaluation of his patient and his theory of therapy. His influence is enhanced by his role and his status, his attitude of concern, and his patient's apprehension about being evaluated."[43]

In short, the so-called epidemic of mental illness is a self-fulfilling prophecy created by the institutional mental-health system. It is an artifact of the set of uniform and limited expectations maintained about individuals who have been psychiatrically labelled—and an artifact of mental health workers' expectations about their own ability to genuinely help individuals who act in socially deviant ways.

The facts reviewed above suggest that the search for the specific genetic defect is otiose. Research demonstrates that environmental factors *cannot* be excluded: there *is* a genetic predisposition to having a breakdown or to becoming psychiatrically labelled. But as noted above, there is reason to suspect that the same kind of genotype constitutes an advantage in other cultures: the individual becomes initiated into the vocation of the shaman. What needs to be changed is not people's genetic codes, but the sensibilities of those who are in positions of power and authority in this society. "The genetic defect myth loses its persuasiveness when we ask, 'By what standard is the individual defective?' As we have seen with the case of 'schizophrenia,' the individual is defective when judged by the standard of modern Western society. But that is no absolute—is an individual to be judged defective because he or she is not predisposed to conform

---

[43]Jerome Frank, *Persuasion and Healing* (New York: Schocken Books, 1973), 127–28

to the current cultural norm? Certainly this individual will face greater obstacles, but this fact may give him or her the impetus to contribute to the transformation of a culture that does not encourage the expansion of the human spirit. The individual with a genetic 'defect' may actually be genetically predisposed to make a greater contribution to the process of spiritual evolution that I believe is taking place on the planet. When viewed from a broader perspective, what is termed a genetic defect may in actuality constitute a genetic opportunity."[44]

There has been one major change in the mental health field in the past 10 years. For decades, 'schizophrenia' had been what Szasz called "the sacred symbol of psychiatry". As Szasz wrote, "The symbol that most specifically characterizes psychiatrists as members of a distinct group of doctors is the concept of schizophrenia; and the ritual that does so most clearly is their diagnosing this disease in persons who do not want to be their patients. . . . Schizophrenia has become the Christ on the cross that psychiatrists worship, in whose name they march in the battle to reconquer reason from unreason, sanity from insanity; reverence toward it has become the mark of psychiatric ortho- doxy, and irreverence toward it the mark of psychiatric here- sy."[45] The new sacred symbol of psychiatry is 'manic- depression', also termed 'bipolar disorder'. People who have breakdowns are now most likely to be told that they suffer from manic-depression, that is to say, a defective metabolic system that has been genetically programmed to become imbalanced at regular or irregular intervals, completely independent of the circumstances in which the individual finds himself or herself.

The number of individuals diagnosed 'schizophrenic' or 'neu- rotic' has dwindled, whereas the number of individuals diag- nosed as 'manic-depressive' has mushroomed,[46] leading the less than wholly credulous observer to the conclusion that the kinds of individuals who were previously diagnosed as 'schizophrenic' or 'neurotic' are now diagnosed as 'manic-depressive'. Manic- depressive associations are springing up everywhere and mental health workers sing reverential praises to Lithium. An individual who has a breakdown is told that he or she has a 'chronic recurrent illness, analogous to diabetes', and that he or she must

[44]Seth Farber, 'The Challenge of Cosmic Optimism', *op. cit.,* 34

[45]Thomas Szasz, *Schizophrenia: The Sacred Symbol of Psychiatry* (New York: Basic Books, 1976), xiv

[46]Lee Coleman, *The Reign of Error* (Boston: Beacon Press, 1984), 149–150

accept the ingestion of lithium carbonate for the rest of his or her life.

This prognosis becomes a self-fulfilling prophecy. As the diagnosis of 'schizophrenia' is irreversible so is the diagnosis of 'manic-depression'. Two of the major promoters of Lithium, for example, described a number of cases where individuals stopped taking Lithium and actually felt better. The pleasant feelings that these individuals experienced were described by the promoters of Lithium as "pathological". They described a writer: "She finally discontinued the lithium carbonate therapy and is now finishing her next novel which her editors state appears very favorable. She's now relaxed, comfortable, happy, and says that for the first time in a long time she's really enjoying life. She remains at present in a mild hypo-manic state."[47] Thus, to paraphrase the old adage, the bland use all their powers to persuade the unbland to come to them in order to be made bland.

After 16 years of studying psychology, after many years of working as a psychotherapist in clinics and later in private practice, after many years of listening to people's stories, I am convinced there's no such entity as mental illness and that as long as we attempt to comprehend individuals with the use of the categories provided by the mental health establishment, we will injure them. The mental health establishment has snowed the American people: it launches the most unimaginably brutal psychological and physical assault on human beings in distress, calls this 'medical treatment', and then blames the outcome on 'mental illness'.

This book argues that the mental health establishment is wrong. It will not, of course, demonstrate this to those who do not have the ears to hear. For these individuals, 'schizophrenia' is a chronic disease and I am just another naive romanticist who does not understand the complexity of the problems of the severely mentally ill.

I am indeed arguing that the majority of individuals labelled 'chronically mentally ill' would become creative individuals and responsible citizens if treated with sensitivity, compassion, and intelligence—if encouraged. I believe this on the basis both of my experience of working with people who are psychiatrically labelled and of my readings. A small group are perhaps more

---

[47]Quoted in Breggin, *Psychiatric Drugs: Hazards to the Brain, op. cit.,* 200

intractable. Individuals who commit violent crimes, like Charles Manson, are associated in the popular mind with the 'mentally ill'. It should be noted, however, that these individuals are criminals, not patients. Violent crimes are less common among people who have been in psychiatric hospitals than among the 'normal' population. Statistically, a person labelled 'mental patient' is *less* likely to commit a violent attack than someone not so labelled.

It is undeniable, of course, that individuals do experience problems in life and that they frequently act in ways that are not conducive to their own emotional and spiritual well-being and development. If this were not the case there would be no need for therapy at all. It is not that they are 'mentally ill' or defective; they simply do not possess the wisdom, skills, or trust in the environment that would enable them to resolve, without guidance, the particular life challenges that confront them as individuals. The role of the therapist is not to eradicate an illness but to provide guidance, direction, emotional support, and encouragement to persons who are involved in a process of learning and growth.

My hope is that the testimony recorded in this book will make it more likely for an individual to get up and walk away when the psychiatrist, psychologist or social worker he or she is consulting says, 'You have a chronic mental illness'. Walk away because this statement is an insult to your dignity as a human being, and lacks any scientific foundation. It is time to say 'No' to the mental health establishment. It is time to put an end to the horrific nightmare they have created.

CHAPTER TEN

Rejecting 'Mental Illness': An Interview with James Mancuso

Farber: One of the theses of your book is that there is no such thing as mental illness.

Mancuso: Mental illness is a concept used to characterize behavior that is unwanted. It exists in the mind of the person who uses the concept to categorize others.

Farber: The term 'mental illness' denotes an interpretation.

Mancuso: Absolutely, one which is unwarranted by the evidence, by the sensibility and by the criteria of what makes a good story. It does not make a good story to say that people who behave in these ways are mentally ill.

Farber: In your book it is shown that despite popular opinions the researchers in psychology have not succeeded in showing that 'schizophrenics' are essentially different from other human beings.

Mancuso: Yes. And the clearest evidence of that is that when someone currently does a study of so-called schizophrenics, nobody takes any indicator, any dependent variable from past work, to use as a criterion for schizophrenia in the process of setting up the experimental group. They still take recourse to relying upon the diagnosis given the person by the psychiatrists. Since the person is typically given different diagnoses by various psychiatrists, the researcher will take the one chosen by a majority of the diagnosers. Obviously, the category is in the mind of the categorizer. Thus, no one yet has found a way

James Mancuso has been professor of psychology at the State University of New York of Albany since 1961. He is the author of numerous articles and author or editor of six books.

	to say, 'Let's use this external criterion that has been found valid.'
Farber:	What the research is really trying to do is to demonstrate that so-called schizophrenics are inferior.
Mancuso:	Yes. Exactly. In our book we make it clear that every hypothesis about schizophrenia attributes inferiority to that state. We make the statement, for example, that a higher body temperature (which has been attributed to schizophrenics) might be a superior condition. When you have an invasion of bacteria, your temperature goes up and helps eliminate the bacteria so this could be a physically beneficial state.
Farber:	Do you agree with the Laingian idea that people who are psychotic are more sensitive?
Mancuso:	People who have been through this experience would be more likely to accept that there are an infinite number of ways of construing events. I think Western society has consistently promulgated the idea that there is one correct way of construing events and some of us happen to be superior construers. The people whom we label as schizophrenic—we are intent on demonstrating that they are inferior construers because that allows us to continue with this search for a disease.
Farber:	Construing people in such a way that we diminish their life choices is not an ethical venture. Do you agree?
Mancuso:	Yes. That is an ethical position that I would take as a person.
Farber:	How did you come to have such an unusual perspective as a psychologist?
Mancuso:	I grew up as a Veterans Administration-trained clinical psychologist at the University of Rochester where the prevalent approach was psychoanalytic. There were also a number of behaviorists. I worked for two years as a school psychologist. Almost by accident I stumbled over George Kelly's psychology of personal

construction. I was looking in the card cata-
logue for Piaget's book *The Construction of
Personal Reality* and I ran across *The Psychology of Personal Constructs*. After that I could
not revert to the notion that people are passive
respondents to an active environment. The
person is an active respondent to an active
environment and the activity that goes on as
the person responds is the construing and
reconstruing of the input that the person is
receiving.

Farber: The psychoanalysts and the behaviorists agreed
that schizophrenics were inferior.

Mancuso: There is no doubt about it.

Farber: How does Kelly's theory relate to working with
people who get themselves put in mental hospitals?

Mancuso: If we go along with the basic tenet of constructive
alternativism we will realize that there are an
infinite number of ways of construing input.
We do not have a mind-free reality. Knowledge
exists within a system of meaning. My knowledge is arcane and meaningless to someone
who does not make contact with the kinds of
constructions and meanings that I generally
use when interpreting events. No one should
be engaging in science if they are unaware of
their own epistemological positions. That's the
problem with modern psychology. We go after
people who are different and refuse to understand that their statements may make sense in
the context of their system of constructions.
We chopped out their brains, dumped toxic
drugs into their bodies, and we justified it all
on the basis of this mental-illness concept.
This is antithetical to accomplishing the task
that needs to be accomplished: to help these
people to develop a positive identity.

Farber: What you are talking about is what you called a
contextualist approach.

Mancuso: Absolutely. The context for understanding has to include the response to the self-definition.

Farber: The professionals respond to the mental patients's self-definition by completely contesting it and getting them to accept a degraded social identity.

Mancuso: The professional who accepts the concept of mental illness is going to degrade the person. That is basically the *object* of the mental-health world.

Farber: Why do you think professionals are so inflexible?

Mancuso: There is a huge power structure supporting the concept of mental illness. At Albany State we have a guy who is totally tied in with the people who are writing the new version of *The Diagnostic and Statistical Manual of Mental Disorders.* If you were a graduate student and saw Mancuso writing the esoteric stuff that he does and this guy working on *DSM IV,* who would you think would help your career move? It's a huge system of support. Whoever controls the development of knowledge has tremendous power. They determine who will or will not get tenure—and that decision is based on factors other than the intrinsic scholastic value of a person's work.

CHAPTER ELEVEN

Psychiatry and Social Control: An Interview with Ron Leifer

Leifer: I was trained at Syracuse under Tom Szasz; and I am a colleague of Ernest Becker. We were with Szasz in the early years at Syracuse. In 1969 I went into private practice and have been in private practice since then. In my writings I'm attempting to build a new paradigm for looking at varieties of human suffering in a way which empowers people rather than disempowers them, which helps people to understand their lives as opposed to being managed by other people, so they can take responsibility for themselves, that is, to find some kind of guiding images which enable them to take responsibility for their own behavior and conduct of life and also for their own experiences, including their own suffering of various kinds, by whatever name you want to call it. Psychiatric categories are simply one variety of names among a huge lexicon of names that various forms of human suffering could be called. Since there aren't really any competing models in our society, we think the psychiatric categories are the only ones. But there are many ways of looking at psychological suffering which integrate the experience, whatever it is, of depression or anxiety; and also help to enlighten the individual about the nature of the relation between the inner world and the outer world; and facilitate an increasing mastery over the inner world, the outer world, and how to bridge the two.

Farber: Like Szasz, you agree that the use of so-called disease

Ron Leifer, M.D., has been a psychiatrist in private practice for over 20 years. He is the author of *In The Name of Mental Health* (New York: Science House, 1969), and numerous articles.

categories, disease metaphors, prevents that from
taking place.

Leifer: That's one of the reasons why I'm critical of the
medical model, because I think the disease categories disempower people and prevent people
from understanding themselves and taking responsibility for themselves. Rather, the concept
of mental illness promotes the power of an elite
few who profess to have secret or esoteric knowledge, and their relationship to society is unclear
and unspoken. Their function is to manage people. Nobody dares speak about it; that's forbid-
den. That's the relationship between psychiatry
and society, and the social function of psychiatry.
Most psychiatrists pretend psychiatry has no social function, it's just a medical discipline. So if
you ask them what the social functions are, they
look at you quizzically. You would never ask
what the social functions of medicine are—
they're to help people who have diseases recover
from their illnesses.

Farber: So you're seeing this historically, psychiatry originat-
ing in the desire on the part of society to deal
with people who weren't conforming to the social
order.

Leifer: Yes and whose non-conformity fell outside the law's
jurisdiction because they were not breaking the
law. In other words, if somebody is a non-con-
formist and breaks the law, then the law will take
care of them. But we can't have a society which
claims to be a free society where the laws are so
restrictive that they criminalize certain styles of
speech and conduct. So you need a supplemen-
tary form of social control which can regulate
styles and forms of conduct which the law can't
regulate.

Farber: And, which is to contrast the social control function
of psychiatry with the idea of therapy: helping
people, empowering people, to deal with the
problems of life, so that one would have to say
that those people who are therapists are a small
minority compared to those people who are just

doing what you just described.

Leifer: In the early sixties a fermentation began to occur, an interdisciplinary fermentation between psychoanalysis, anthropology, sociology, psychology, and political science. People from these disciplines were being brought to Syracuse because of the broad orientation of Szasz and Hollander.

Farber: I didn't know that Hollander was at all an iconoclast.

Leifer: Actually, the interdisciplinary confluence began prior to 1960 with the previous chairman, Edward Stainbrook, who is a professor emeritus at UCLA. When he was chairman, he established liaisons, particularly with the department of anthropology. That was in 1953.

Farber: O.K. so it looked like changes were taking place in psychoanalysis itself, you're saying, right?

Leifer: Well, it wasn't that. It was that psychoanalysis had a tremendous impact on American intellectual life, especially in New York City, but also in Chicago. It had an influence on anthropology, English literature, and psychology, so that psychoanalysis, which was alive and thriving at the time, was energizing all these other disciplines, and *vice versa.* And at Syracuse in particular, these things were coming together because of Ed Stainbrook, and Hollander, and Szasz, who followed Stainbrook.

Farber: And one of the implications of this is that they started looking for social explanations of behavior that had previously been thought to be a result of individual malfunctioning?

Leifer: No, actually it was more of an addendum to psychoanalysis, that is taking Freud's rather narrow view and expanding it with new approaches from the social sciences. This was prior to the time that the social sciences got taken over by the computer people.

Farber: This was not an attempt to find social explanations of deviant behavior?

Leifer: Well, it was because one of the fruits of this cross-fertilization between psychiatry and the social sciences was Ernie Becker, who was very broadly educated in the social sciences, and who wrote the book *Revolution and Psychiatry* in which he attempts to re-interpret schizophrenia and depression from a broad psychological, psycho-anthropological point of view. At the same time Szasz was writing critically of psychiatry, and I myself, then a junior member, was pumping in a few articles. I wrote an article on phobia, some articles on psychiatry and the law, and of course, our students were becoming drawn into this. The conservative psychiatrists at the medical school could see this new force growing, which would have been, had it grown, an alternative to the current biological psychiatry. Psychiatry was then at a crossroads, because it was crossing into the social sciences and getting further and further away from medicine. So there was a counter-reaction, to bring psychiatry back into medicine, in order to, first of all, support the social identity of psychiatrists as physicians.

Farber: They undermine the hegemony of psychiatrists within the profession if they don't insist that social problems are medical diseases.

Leifer: Exactly. This, then, requires them to find biological explanations for 'mental illness'.

Farber: Which is exactly what they're trying to do now.

Leifer: Yes! And these biological explanations help circumvent Szasz's critique. The conservative psychiatrists attempted to neutralize this group of people who were working on an alternative approach to problems in mental health.

Farber: Psychoanalysts, if anything, have now made their peace with biological psychiatry.

Leifer: That's right. Psychoanalysts have made their compromise with biological psychiatry. But back then, there was a tremendous energy and a potential fruitfulness of the dialogue between psychoanalysis and the social sciences. That social movement got repressed by what happened in Syracuse.

Farber: And whatever intellectual developments have taken

place in that direction have taken places on the margins of psychiatry.

Leifer: On the margins of psychiatry, ignored by psychiatry. Ernie Becker's books were never reviewed. Szasz's books are hardly ever reviewed in the psychiatric literature. I wouldn't say never, but rarely.

Farber: In the textbooks in the sixties and seventies, there were always a few references to Szasz, not complimentary. But now, in the latest editions, they omit any mention of him altogether.

Leifer: Right. This is a kind of, I won't call it a conspiracy, but it's a kind of a common professional identity problem and resolution by simply making Szasz into a non-person and not reading Becker and simply repressing the possibility that the phenomena that we call mental illness can be more broadly viewed as variations on human conduct and experience.

Farber: Without denigrating individuals and labelling them.

Leifer: Without attempting to control people. Just as a scientific description. People go through different experiences and behave differently. They do. And sometimes what they do is disturbing. It is. But the point is that psychiatry should be totally removed from any kind of political action. Social control is definitely political action.

Farber: It's persecution of people with deviant world-views, similar to the persecution of heretics by the Catholic Church.

Leifer: Right. Now, that's where my point comes in, that psychiatry is a covert mechanism of social control. My first book was devoted to explaining why it's covert.

Farber: When people talk about social control, we think of revolutionaries who pose a danger to the State, whereas these individuals didn't pose a danger to the State.

Leifer: Yes, they did.

Farber: People labelled schizophrenic.

Leifer: Of course they do. Listen, this psychiatric movement was used, and I want to make this public, because it's been ignored. It was used to suppress the civil rights movement in the South.

Farber: I didn't know that.

Leifer: I was very active in the civil rights movement, and my black friends from the South told me of many cases of active black civil rights workers who were handled by psychiatry in the South; that was never publicized.

Farber: Well, I guess psychiatrists are willing to get involved in any venture that anyone invites them into.

Leifer: Oh, absolutely. Now they're doing it in the drug war. I saw Rangel on TV the other night. He's the top Eichmann in the drug war—the top executor or henchman or leader of the movement. Just as Eichmann was moving the Jews into the concentration camps, Rangel is moving the druggies into the prisons and mental hospitals. He says that this guy from Stanford who tells students that he used MDMA, and it was to his benefit, ought to be fired from Stanford, and Stanford will be deprived of one hundred million dollars of federal funds because this guy at Stanford is leading impressionable young people to believe there's something valuable in drugs. One of the panelists asks Rangel well, what are the reasons that marijuana is illegal? Rangel says, I don't know, I'm not a doctor. I just believe what the doctors say. He is as impressionable as he accuses this professor from Stanford of being.

Farber: So people get persecuted in many cases for selling or using drugs that are far less dangerous than the drugs that psychiatrists persecute people for not using.

Leifer: You know how many people die from marijuana?

Farber: I presume hardly any.

Leifer: None. You know how many people die from dog bites? Twenty-five per year. Twenty-five people a year are killed by dogs, not by marijuana. And last week you could see on TV cops coming in with guns on people smoking marijuana.

Farber: And then we also have this great public health crisis as a result of tardive dyskinesia caused by the neuroleptic drugs that psychiatrist push.

Leifer: And your experience and my experience of finding plenty of doctors who will put people on these drugs, indeed, force people to take them, and nobody who will take responsibility supervising people getting off. There are more people being damaged by psychiatric drugs than by illegal drugs.

Farber: Yes. Now, Szasz was not, in fact, fired. They just attempted to . . .

Leifer: He had tenure.

Farber: Oh, that's why. They wanted to move him into a different building, which was more or less just an insult, wasn't it?

Leifer: It's not that they wanted to move him into a different building; it's that the chairman of the department had his office in the state hospital. And Koch, the head of the department of mental hygiene of New York State, forbade Szasz from teaching in the hospital because he said his views on mental illness would influence residents into maltreating the patients. Szasz was no longer permitted to teach in the place where the department office was.

Farber: It was coming from the state, you're saying.

Leifer: The order that forbade Szasz from teaching in the Hospital came from the state director of the department of mental hygiene.

Farber: So they were attempting to suppress Szasz.

Leifer: To suppress Szasz, right.

Farber: But they couldn't do it, anyway, because even if he wasn't teaching in the Hospital, he would still be listed in the syllabus, right?

Leifer: Right. They didn't affect his academic appointment. And, in fact, Hollander, at one point, when Szasz boycotted the meetings and Ernie Becker and I also boycotted the meetings, brought this to the attention of the whole department. Some of the people in the department thought that Ernie and I should be fired for, just simply, disobedience.

Hollander was willing to move the meeting to the medical school, but Szasz continued to boycott it so long as there was any connection between the department of mental hygiene and the department of psychiatry. And this split the department down the middle.

Farber: Szasz was obviously objecting to the State intervention . . .

Leifer: Exactly. Szasz was objecting to the department of mental hygiene, which is an office of the State, interfering in the academic affairs . . .

Farber: Academic freedom then, it would be.

Leifer: To me and to Szasz and to Becker it was an attempt to silence Szasz.

Farber: And, at any rate, they did succeed, as you say, in suppressing the movement in general.

Leifer: They did succeed.

Farber: Was it a result of actions like that?

Leifer: No, nobody knew about that. It was the result of Tom's book *The Myth of Mental Illness* being published in 1961. After that, when Becker was fired in 1964 and I was fired in 1966, neither of us could get jobs in psychiatry because of our association with Szasz. So it wasn't just that this was a symbolic act at the medical school; it was simply the beginning of the attempt by psychiatry to negate this whole movement.

Farber: It's amazing when you think of the parallel between them attempting to suppress dissident psychiatrists, how it parallels the attempt to put mental patients in mental hospitals.

Leifer: That's why I say that I'm a victim of psychiatry. Then they call you by psychiatric names. They began to tell unfounded stories about Szasz. To this day, he still has a reputation in psychiatry as being mentally ill. That's how they dismiss him.

Farber: Many of the victims of psychiatry don't present dangers to the State. Are psychiatrists threatened by anyone who deviates from a particular norm?

Leifer: They *all* present dangers to the State because, Seth, what is free speech? I mean, does free speech mean letting a schizophrenic babble on the street corner?

Farber: Certainly it does.

Leifer: But that's why psychiatry abridges the First Amendment.

Farber: But how does that present a danger to the State? I mean, they may certainly present . . .

Leifer: The State is its own internal contradiction. While it believes in all these constitutional rights, it really doesn't want to permit them. And so what it does, it uses psychiatry as a covert means of social control.

Farber: So, the political State has decided it has interests in perpetuating the status quo, or tolerating only certain behaviors.

Leifer: That's right. Now Ezra Pound, was that mental illness or free speech?

Farber: So, you have a State that enforces conformity to norms and is afraid of any degree of deviance from that, even if it doesn't take a political form of threatening to overthrow the State in any sense?

Leifer: It gets down to questions of personal identity. In the fifties Levi-Strauss said that the notion of 'primitive' was based on an idea of westerners who wanted to create a gap between what it meant to be civilized and what it meant to be Third World. In the same way, the concept of 'mental illness' is designed to place a gap between what's normal and what's not normal.

Farber: So society's positing of its own identity requires it to create this stereotype?

Leifer: Exactly. The positing of its own identity. The function of mental illness is to create the boundaries of legitimate identity.

Farber: But I mean this stereotype of the 'other' is created by the very same process in which it defines its own identity. This gives a feeling of security.

Leifer: The creation of one's own identity requires the posit-

ing of a 'not me'. In order to know where the
boundaries of 'me' and 'not me' are. And even
though everybody's thought processes are, you
know, what Freud called 'primary process', we
project that onto the schizophrenic as if only the
schizophrenic has primary process, when the
truth of the matter is that the schizophrenic is
speaking his or her mind, and everybody else has
the same kind of thoughts but keeps them silent
and speaks in a kind of a pro forma dialect.

Farber: Why is that kind of discourse—one might say it's a
discourse, to use a fancy term—the discourse of
dreams or primary process, why is that not
allowed to be spoken?

Leifer: Because it so often strikes at the truths we don't want
to see. Namely, 'Mother, you hate me!' 'Father,
you're a son of bitch!' 'I want to sleep with you!'
It's free speech. It's stating one is being controlled by electricity, while everybody is watching
TV.

Farber: So anyway, what happened in the sixties?

Leifer: A social-intellectual movement was successfully repressed and quashed in order to promote a biological psychiatry which reinforced psychiatric
identity as medical, which got money from the
NIMH, which was cutting down on its funds and
giving money only to legitimate scientific projects, defined as projects which measured and
were objective rather than political or subjective
in any sense. And it made the control of the
population by covert means more invisible by
justifying the actions with medical jargon. If it
stayed on the other side, it would have become
very ideological, and this is now during the period of the civil rights movement and the Vietnam
War, when there was clamping down on the intellectual life of this country. All the Marxists at the
universities who didn't have tenure were expelled
in the sixties.

Farber: You would also link the mental patients liberation
movement up with the Civil Rights movement as

well as movements in Russia, is that true?

Leifer: I would link it. In my experience, the civil rights movement, the anti-war movement and the anti-psychiatry movement were all of one piece in the sixties.

Farber: And you put them in one category with the movements in Russia.

Leifer: The anti-state movements, the national liberation movements in Czechoslovakia and the Soviet Union. All of one piece.

Farber: Both Laing and Szasz were accused of romanticizing, Laing particularly was accused of romanticizing mental illness. Szasz and Laing were both accused of underestimating the terrible suffering that these people go through.

Leifer: I don't think it was Laing who romanticized the mentally ill; I think it was the people who read Laing who romanticized it. What Laing was saying was that psychosis wasn't simply a kind of a passive experience. It was an active experience in which the individual was trying to grope and reconcile the contradictions of reality. So it was in some sense a growth process, and if people were helped to go through this in a way suited to their own rhythms and given a little help along the way, they could come out of it, and it might be some kind of a learning experience. Now, that isn't to say they're necessarily going to come out of it as saints or come out of it as heroes, just simply come out of it with a learning experience. Because Laing, I think, recognized that people do grow and learn as they go through this kind of a very painful experience.

Farber: But you know, Ron, I'd like to make the point that the psychiatrists have de-romanticized virtually every dimension of human existence, or they have attempted to do so. Max Weber wrote about the industrial revolution and the "disenchantment" and rationalization of the world. This is merely another aspect of this process. It's only in the last couple of hundred years that madness has

been defined as a medical disease. Madness has
always had a tremendous romantic allure and a
mystique for the artist, the poet, the romantic. It
goes back to Shakespeare, and even before that,
to Plato. I maintain that the mad person has
pierced the veil of illusion, and has seen something that 'normal' people frequently do not see.
And I do not believe that madness has to be so
very painful. The problem, even before the mad
person starts being tortured by psychiatrists, is
that there is no one to talk this language with, no
one to commune with. It's like he or she is a
Martian on the planet Earth—and it's that loneliness that is so terribly frightening. You know if
you're having an LSD trip and you commune
with God and all around you are a bunch of
squares who negate the existence of any reality of
spirit, who see you just as a nut, it's frightening
and lonely. And I think that is what Laing was
trying to point out. If we as a culture accepted
madness it would not be so frightening for the
individual.

Leifer: You're probably right. Which brings me to the second
point. I know that Szasz was not oblivious to the
fact that people suffer, but he thought suffering
was a part of life, and that to deprive people of
their freedom because they were suffering was to
compound the tragedy. It's no help to people who
are suffering to deprive them of their freedom.
We won't even release the names of people who
have AIDS. Why do we treat people who we say
are mentally ill and deprive them of their freedom? This is obviously political.

Farber: The same argument goes back to Dostoevski's Grand
Inquisitor. The Grand Inquisitor promises people
that he'll deliver them happiness and security. All
they have to turn over is their freedom.

Leifer: That's the same thing. Szasz was not oblivious to
people's suffering. On the contrary. He knew very
well about suffering, having himself fled from
antisemitic Hungary at the age of 19 and come to
this country as an immigrant, and gone through

painful enough experiences himself, with his family health and what not. He is not a man who is oblivious or insensitive to suffering. It's just that his values go beyond the so-called compassion which psychiatrists profess, but hypocritically.

Farber: Szasz said, and Laing had said the same thing, that in order to help a person you first have to feel a sense of kinship with that person.

Leifer: Right.

Farber: Now, these psychoanalysts who write the books on empathy and all that—that's very popular in psychoanalytic circles—they're the first to lock someone up, they're the first to give them electroshock. You can't feel a sense of empathy with someone you've defined as a chronic schizophrenic, a schizotypal disorder.

Leifer: Absolutely true. So that this claim that Szasz was indifferent to people's suffering is a projection.

Farber: And so what you have then, you have not compassion or empathy, but you have perhaps a sympathy tinged with contempt and revulsion, which seems to me the essence of pity.

Leifer: I think you have basically self-interested indifference to people.

Farber: Do you want to say what you've done over the years to help people in distress and how that's changed as a result of your meeting Szasz and your reading Laing?

Leifer: The view I've come to is that psychotherapy is basically a spiritual process in which people come with pain, and it's not, for the most part, a pain that's caused by anything going on in their body. It's caused by the way in which they relate to life. And the way in which people relate to life fundamentally has been addressed by religion. Now, I myself am a Buddhist . . .

Farber: And you became a Buddhist in . . .

Leifer: I became a Buddhist in 1979. I took my vows then, although I had meditation training from the early sixties. It became clear to me that the oriental

religions, particularly Buddhism, Hinduism, and
Taoism, had so much to say about the nature of
mind and the nature of suffering that, after psychoanalysis had basically exhausted itself and
psychiatry had turned biological, I turned myself
towards the oriental religions for understanding
the mind. And particularly Buddhism. And from
Buddhism I discovered certain principles which I
have found very helpful not only in my own life
but in counseling people who are suffering mental, psychological, emotional distress. And so I
try without labelling it as Buddhism or being in
any way overtly religious, to use these principles
in order to help people out of their own traps.

Farber: And it works?

Leifer: It's not that it works, it's that when somebody takes
it and applies it, it works.

Farber: What are the main principles?

Leifer: The main principle is that our suffering is caused by
our desires.

Farber: And do you want to state how you put that into
practice with a client?

Leifer: Well, for example, if somebody comes in with anger
as a problem I discuss this with them. The formula for anger is that somebody has a desire,
that is, 'I want this or I don't want that', the
desire is frustrated by some kind of obstacle, external or internal, then the result of the frustration of the desire is the feeling of helplessness
and fear. The response to that helplessness and
fear is anger. Anger is a biological response to
danger. The feeling of helplessness is the feeling
of being in danger. It was created by wanting
something that we can't have. That makes us feel
as if we're helpless and vulnerable. The anger is a
kind of a physiological response to that helplessness, and its psychological function is to oblite-
rate the sensation of helplessness and
vulnerability. When somebody thinks they can
get what they want or avoid what they don't
want, their energy will be anger energy. If they
themselves don't feel it's possible to get it, either

because of external circumstances or because they lack their own resources or willingness, they begin to feel hopeless. And that combination of hopelessness and helplessness is depression. But it all starts with the desires. So that in order for a person who is angry or depressed to help themselves, they have to come to an awareness of their own desires and how those desires are frustrated and how that frustration leads them to a state of hopelessness and helplessness. Fundamentally you might call it psycho-spiritual—there's no difference between psychological and spiritual.

Farber: But isn't it legitimate to help that person realize their desires?

Leifer: Of course. It's a fundamental education. But that's why psychotherapy is more like an educational enterprise than it is like a medical enterprise. But spiritual therapy can be either a kind of a ministering an active agent to a passive recipient or it can be an induction of the person's own resources by somebody who's skillful in inducing people to begin to operate more effectively themselves in behalf of their own happiness.

Farber: Are you saying also then that being aware of this, one can attain clarity that will allow one not to be overwhelmed by feelings of helplessness?

Leifer: Yes.

Farber: And that would enable one to attain what is in fact attainable and to renounce the accomplishment of what's outside of one's powers?

Leifer: Yes, I can accept that. In fact, you might say that the function of therapy is to help people to achieve this awareness and practice the skills in approaching life in a way that's rational and skillful as opposed to awkward and self-defeating.

Farber: And, now, people who have consulted you who would be considered by the psychiatric Establishment to be severely mentally ill, or schizophrenic—you've found that you're able to help these people and help them stay out of mental hospitals?

Leifer: Yes, especially if they have a supportive network flexible enough to enter into dialogue. Some people will *only* accept the medical model. Those people I feel sorry for, because I think it's disempowering.

Farber: I want to bring it back to more positive experiences that are suppressed by the mental health system that are frequently associated with the phenomenon that they label 'schizophrenia'.

Leifer: Well, you know, culture and art and literature and music are all the product of mentation. So that obviously mentation isn't all bad unless you're going to be a Buddhist monk. But it's also possible to have too much of a good thing. And there are people whose minds are so hyperactive and unproductive, that on balance the experience for them is negative.

Farber: Well, it's also a question then of knowing when to control it, or be able to turn it on and turn it off.

Leifer: What I say to people is, you've already got the 'On' switch; now you need an 'Off' switch. And you have to be in control of the 'On' switch and the 'Off' switch.

Farber: I think that one of the problems in this society, particularly in the mental health system is that these therapists suffer from a poverty of imagination.

Leifer: Well, we have to be careful of our language. You know, hypermentation can be very narrow. And just simply go over again and again the same old tracks.

Farber: I was identifying something different. I wasn't thinking of hypermentation in that sense. I was thinking of someone with all these fantasies and unusual associations.

Leifer: They can be creative.

Farber: Well, Laing made the point and I've certainly seen it, that people who get psychiatrically labelled more frequently than not seem to be poetically minded.

Leifer: Well, I would say, and I know that Szasz would say, because we've discussed this before, that they speak in poetry. As a matter of fact, Becker's term for this was, you might say his synonym for schizophrenia was, 'Homo poetica'.

Farber: As Shakespeare says, "the lunatic, the lover, and the poet are of imagination all compact."

Leifer: Well, schizophrenia and poetry are both products of mentation. And in the schizophrenic's mentation there is some poetry. And in the poet's poetry there is some hypermentation. So, it depends. You know, there's certain poetry I don't enjoy. On the other hand, I don't think I've ever met anyone in a mental hospital who I couldn't talk to. So, I think if you have a poetic mind, you can talk to anybody.

Farber: Laing always said he felt far more of a sense of kinship with the person locked up in the mental hospital than he did with the psychiatrist who does the locking up. He said he felt on the other side of that great divide.

Leifer: Me too.

Farber: And psychiatrists tend to talk—I think Szasz has demonstrated this pretty clearly—they tend to talk in these clichés, and these banalities, that they repeat over and over again.

Leifer: Sure.

Farber: You would agree that most so-called psychotic people are much more interesting?

Leifer: Absolutely. Far more imaginative. Far more present-centered. Far more in touch with life. But I don't want to be accused of glamorizing the state because I don't think it's a particularly intelligent state. I don't think it's particularly intelligent to be locked up in a mental hospital.

Farber: No, not to be locked up.

Leifer: You know, if somebody gets themselves to that point and is not able to get out, there's a certain lack of intelligence. It's generally easy to get out of a mental hospital.

Farber: I had someone who got out of a mental hospital, and I let her stay in my apartment. She'd walked out, and they hadn't made any attempt to get her back. I didn't let her stay long, but a few days. She was in a state of distress but she wasn't freaked out. She wasn't having anything that would be characterized as a breakdown. She sat in my living room, and I didn't have time to talk to her, and she was: blah blah blah blah. She said: 'Well, I'll talk to your cat or I'll talk to the wall'. She sat there for three hours talking to herself until she was calm.

Leifer: No, but Seth, if you were this woman's husband or mother or father you might not be able to tolerate it. But you wouldn't want to kick her out, you'd want to appear to be compassionate and helpful. So you'd refer her to a psychiatrist who calls her mentally ill and gets her out. You've got her out, and you don't have to see yourself as a bad person.

Farber: But all I had to teach her to do was to talk to herself rather than attempt to talk to someone else.

Leifer: That's true.

Farber: Occasionally I would respond to her, but I stopped doing it and attended to my own work. So when I ignored her, she realized she was not going to get my attention, and she discovered that just talking to *herself* filled a function for her.

Leifer: I understand what you're saying, but there's another side to it also. And that is, if you were married to her, you'd probably want a divorce. And if she couldn't take care of herself, there'd be a big problem.

Farber: But also, Ron, there is yet another side to it. You see, her monologue was quite entertaining. She had developed a sense of humor, so it was difficult at times to ignore her because there was an element of humor, and even social satire. And of course there was also pain there. So it was easy for me to get lured into listening. But I didn't because I had work to do. And also, I trusted that however much pain she had she could handle it on her own. But the mental health people could not see her charms, or character, or acknowledge then, because they had to filter her being through this concept of mental illness. Nor could they see that the solution was to allow her to talk to herself, and to teach others that they need not feel they need to rush in to rescue her. There was some kind of positive value in her learning that she didn't need to tell another person everything that was in her mind, but she could speak it out to herself and somehow that would be a way of calming herself.

Leifer: Just that kind of conversation can be crucially helpful to a person like that. That you don't have to tell other people, you can take a space for yourself and talk it out to yourself, because if you bother people, they'll get irritated with you, they'll call you mentally ill, they'll not want to hurt you, and they'll think they're helping you by putting you . . .

Farber: That's why she was in a mental hospital for so long, just for saying what was on her mind.

Leifer: A very helpful conversation. That's what I would count as psychotherapy.

CHAPTER TWELVE

Getting Off Psychiatric Drugs: An Interview with Ron Leifer

Leifer: When somebody comes in to me to get off drugs, the first thing I explain to them is that the basic reason they're on drugs is that their behavior either doesn't satisfy or disturbs some people around them. So that if they're going to get off drugs, a part of getting off drugs is reducing the demand that other people make that they be on drugs. And in order to do that, they have to take some increased responsibility for their own behavior. So that getting off drugs goes hand in hand with learning something about oneself so that one becomes more skilled at dealing with people and doesn't get into a circumstance where you're being corralled and put on the spot and forced to take drugs basically for other people's benefit.

Farber: I was thinking of the situation Kate Millett describes. It's typical that when a person goes off drugs the people around them generally are people who have accepted the psychiatric version of reality, and so they're going to panic.

Leifer: Well, not only that. They're probably genuinely bothered by her behavior. That is, I think that she has to make some kind of an inquiry into what it is about the way she was conducting herself that frightened people. Now maybe she thought it was exciting and maybe she had a more open attitude towards life and maybe she had more honesty about her inner feelings. All of those things can threaten people. In a certain sense, in order to be 'healthy' and deal with people, you have to be sort of a closed, constricted person.

Farber: So what would you advise someone to do who gets

160

off drugs and finds themselves, not in dangerous situations, but feeling more enthusiastic about life?

Leifer: The first thing that they have to understand is that while to them, to a manic or hypo-manic person, their behavior feels not only appropriate but exhilarating, not everybody may feel that way about their behavior. And the people closest to them may actually be put off by their energy in the same way that parents who love a child can be put off by the energy of the child, if the child is just too full of life. Now another way of describing somebody who is too full of life is 'hyperactive'. But there is something in addition to being too full of life about hyperactivity, and that is the inability to hold one's attention for prolonged periods of time on one stated task rather than flitting from thing to thing. And those people who hold power in society tend to be productive enough, they have that power precisely because they have that power of concentration, and are able to hold themselves to a task. So that holding oneself to a task becomes a socially valued skill, and people who don't have that skill are devalued by these other people who hold power.

Farber: Are you saying that a lot of people who get labelled manic-depressive, for example, haven't developed this skill to . . .

Leifer: To control themselves.

Farber: To hold attention to a particular task?

Leifer: That may be one feature of it. If it's very manic that may be one feature. But it's more that they haven't learned to control their enthusiasm, you might say. But it's not only just to control their enthusiasm, because it's deeper than that. It's understanding that one's basic relationship to life is psychothymic. You know, there are all these categories: dysthymic depression, and psychothymic depression, and tendencies toward psychothymia. Everybody has a tendency toward psychothymia, by which is meant, everybody experiences both highs and lows. There's nobody who doesn't.

Farber: Right. That's obscured by this whole rhetoric about bipolar disorders.

Leifer: It's obscured by this whole thing. Everybody experiences ups and downs. They skim over this when they talk about things like normal mourning versus pathological mourning, or normal variations in mood versus pathological variations in mood. They don't talk about that subject because there are, in reality, only two criteria of pathology in the mental health field, and they are: one, that a person's behavior, thought, or feelings disturbs them . . .

Farber: Disturbs the psychiatrist?

Leifer: Disturbs them themselves; or, two, that their behavior, thought, and the way they express their thought and feelings disturbs the people around them. Those are the only two criteria for pathology. Now those criteria are obscured and they're buried. But if you're willing to inquire deeply enough as to what the fundamental epistemological basis of these psychiatric categories are, they're basically evaluative. The same is true in medicine, by the way, namely that the criteria for disease are: bodily changes cause disease only if they lead to death, disability, or pain. If they don't then they're called normal variations.

Farber: But there you have an ultimately biological criterion.

Leifer: Well, it's not only that it's biological but that they're universally valued. To avoid death, disability, and pain is universally valued.

Farber: Anyway, so you don't have a biological criterion for what they call 'mental pathology' because being disturbed doesn't mean that one has a disease that could lead to death.

Leifer: Right. We're talking here about happiness, we're talking about satisfaction. And there's some cultural variability about that, there's an historical variability within the same society from time to time, whether sexual orientation is a disease or not a

disease. Psychiatrists are constantly inventing new diseases and abandoning their old
diseases.

Farber: It's also this kind of notion, as Szasz says, that people
are supposed to be happy all the time, that there
are not obstacles to the realizations of their aspirations. So if they're not happy they're presumed
to be abnormal.

Leifer: The rule is unhappiness. Happiness is the exception.
But it's this sort of naive psychiatric expectation.
No psychiatrist that I know of today talks about
'normal unhappiness'! From the theoretical point
of view that's a glaring inconsistency which needs
to be paid attention to, namely: why don't psychiatrists talk about ordinary unhappiness? And
what is the difference between ordinary unhappiness and extraordinary unhappiness? Freud was
puzzled by that one.

Farber: My point of view is that one doesn't need to posit
any kind of defect within a person.

Leifer: There are moral defects.

Farber: Yes, moral shortcomings, or whatever.

Leifer: Shortcomings. The exception would be that I think
there is something valid to the biological approach in that we all come endowed with different physical equipment. And there are probably
general features of the physical equipment which
differ among groups. For example, in temperament, which I would think would be something
the neurobiologists would want to explore so that
they could avoid all the complications of mental
illness and psychiatric politics and just simply
explore the biological basis for different physical
temperament, which is obviously genetic.

Farber: Well, that's a whole other question.

Leifer: It's not a whole other question, because it really is
one of the intuitive foundations of modern biological psychiatry.

Farber: It seems that the main thrust of all the biological
research they're doing now is to try to establish

that certain groups of people are inferior to other human beings.

Leifer: Well, there's one other motive. Namely, that psychiatrists have a large field of bigger and bigger business. Psychiatry is a boom industry, which is like oil explorers of old striking gushers in every field that they drilled. Psychiatrists are just finding— actually inventing—more and more mental illnesses.

Farber: I read that in the last 20 years the number of illnesses in the *DSM III* has doubled.

Leifer: More than doubled. Now recently they're saying that for every addiction there's a deficient neurotransmitter. Addiction is no longer a moral problem. They've redefined it as a physical problem and it's in their arena. They're now the experts and the specialists. They're going to get the money, they're going to have more power than all the other mental health professionals. There's an old Zen expression, 'Small person makes self bigger by chopping off heads of others'. Psychiatry, which was threatened during the 1950s by the encroachment of the social sciences, felt small and is now making itself bigger by chopping off the heads of everybody and saying that all behavior now falls under their domain as a form of mental illness.

Farber: And for every illness there's a drug.

Leifer: There are basically three types of psychiatric medications. The first type is aimed at fear. Those are the so-called anti-anxiety drugs, the major and the minor, you know, from Thorazine to Valium and Xanax. On the one hand you have the heavy ones, which are used to control people who are florid in their deviations from the norm, like Mellaril and Stelazine . . .

Farber: In my discussions with people, not a single one of them describes the drug as alleviating their fear or distress.

Leifer: That's a very interesting fact which ought to be publicized. Although there are so-called 'paradoxical reactions', that is, when you feel your freedom is being restricted by a drug you could become more afraid rather than less afraid. But I don't think that the reactions of people who are given these drugs are given enough publicity or credence either by the profession or the public. It's basically ignored as to what it's like to be on these drugs. Nobody cares or nobody talks about that as long as the conduct is brought into line with whatever situation the person is expected to conform to.

Farber: Of course, Breggin says that neuroleptics produce a lobotomy-like effect, they produce an indifference to the environment and a lack of motivation.

Leifer: Yes, and all those things which we spend billions of dollars to prevent people taking, for example, marijuana, supposedly have the same effect. And then we simultaneously spend billions of dollars to force these other drugs upon people.

Farber: Well, marijuana has a pleasant effect on people, too, whereas . . .

Leifer: Something that none of these drugs have. Yet we spend billions of dollars to prevent people from using marijuana and on the other hand force a whole population of other people to take these other drugs which have no redeeming effects and which are quite dangerous.

Farber: You started to say that getting off these drugs involves an increased responsibility.

Leifer: Let me talk about the three categories of drugs: those designed to interfere with the physiology of fear; the psychic energizers or antidepressants, which have the opposite effect of actually activating that fear system; and the Lithium which . . . nobody knows how it works but it's designed for mania and we'll talk about that in a separate group. So, first I'll talk about the anti-anxiety drugs or tranquilizers. Basically, they are necessary for dealing with fear. So what the individual needs to do to get off those drugs.

Farber: Now you're talking about Thorazine, Stelazine, . . .

Leifer: Thorazine, Stelazine, all of those drugs, including

Valium and Xanax.

Farber: I would make a distinction because everyone that I
          interviewed hated Thorazine and Stelazine.

Leifer: Well, they're used primarily to control people's be-
          havior. To me they're the equivalent of PCP in
          the human realm. PCP we use for animals we
          want to knock down because they're dangerous,
          then bring them to a zoo. The same with hu-
          mans. You knock them down with these drugs,
          put them in a cage, and then they're under con-
          trol. But the Valium and the Xanax many people
          ask for and want.

Farber: There's a black market for Valium. You're not going
          to find a black market for Prolixin.

Leifer: Right. And there are a couple of reasons for that.
          And the reason, by the way, there's a black mar-
          ket for Valium, probably, is that it works on the
          same enzyme system as alcohol, so that it proba-
          bly has some of the same pleasant effects as alco-
          hol. It's the gamma system, gamma aminobuturic
          acid. But for a person to deal with fear, the first
          thing I do is say, 'All right. Now we're contract-
          ing to help you get off these drugs that you're on.
          So the first thing I want to do is for you to try a
          graduated reduction schedule. Whatever you're
          on, we're going to lower it by a very small but
          significant amount each week. And we're going to
          go very conservatively, a week at a time, to see
          how you feel and how you behave.' Whatever
          you're on, I would, let's say, cut it by an eighth.
          And then at the same time, teach the person how
          to deal with fear by teaching them how to relax.
          So I do very intensive body relaxation work.
          Physical relaxation cuts the cybernetic anxiety
          pathway. When I say 'cybernetic', it's a feedback
          system. You can get the anxiety system working
          without the anxiety but physiologically exactly
          the same by going for a run. Your heart will
          speed up, your aspiration will increase, the same
          —it's the fight/flight reaction. Running is flight
          without fear. But you can have fear without
          flight. It's the same system that needs to be

turned off. And that system can be turned off simply by relaxing. When you run you're activating the system by basically telling the system: 'The muscles need to be used; start the adrenalin going'. And when you relax the muscles, you're basically telling the body: 'There's no danger, there's no need for action, turn off the whole fight/flight response'.

Farber: I imagine just getting in bed might induce a state of relaxation.

Leifer: Yes, a lot of things will. Taking a bath will. And that's one of the reasons that people take a certain category of drugs, namely, alcohol, marijuana, opiates, you know. Those drugs basically help people to relax. In every society from the beginning of human history there has been some substance used by people to help them relax. Why? Because society creates tension.

Farber: And people also take substances to produce altered states of consciousness.

Leifer: That's a different motivation. This is one basic motivation for using mind-altering substances—to relax.

Farber: I presume a lot of people who read this will not find psychiatrists who agree to take them off Thorazine or Stelazine, so they're going to have to do it on their own.

Leifer: I wouldn't say they're going to have to do it on their own. I mean, they could do it on their own. It's more hazardous, because it's helpful to have a trained person who can help you to make whatever necessary adjustments you have to make.

Farber: I haven't been able to find more than one person— and he's not even seeing anyone now. I've taken people off drugs, just because they trust my authority. But I haven't found one psychiatrist in the New York City area who's willing to help a person gradually get off psychiatric drugs.

Leifer: I would predict that there are as many psychiatrists in New York willing to help people get off drugs as there are DEA agents who use drugs. The propaganda for psychiatry is: 'These drugs are good and should be used; nobody should be off them'. And the propaganda of the DEA is: 'These drugs are bad and should not be used by anybody'. And in each group you have a small minority who violate the rule.

Farber: A person who's gotten a label, 'schizophrenic', and has been in a mental hospital five or six times is likely to have a hard time finding a psychiatrist who's going to agree to get them off Prolixin or whatever.

Leifer: True. They may need a non-professional advisor, which is why it's a good idea for this kind of information to be disseminated as widely as possible, because it's possible to train non-professionals to help other people reduce their psychiatric medication. If psychiatrists won't do it, then maybe some indigenous group of healers can arise who will be down-to-earth enough and educated enough to be able to do this in a skillful manner.

Farber: Well, what Kate Millett did eventually was, she got two ex-mental patients, who had been activists in the mental patient liberation movement—they were the only two people that she told about it and they were people who had themselves gotten off psychiatric drugs.

Leifer: So they could help her.

Farber: Yes, just give her the reassurance and all. Another thing, what she didn't do was tell the other people around her that she was not taking her Lithium. She led them to believe that she was still taking her Lithium, so they wouldn't get frightened.

Leifer: That will work as long as she doesn't annoy them. Let's go to the next step, because this is very important. There's nowhere that this is discussed, so let's cover it. The first thing is to help people relax their body. The second thing is to help them to work with their own mind in a very active way; that is, to actually look at their minds and work with them. And what they have to look at, basically, the basic problem is what I called hypermentation, too much thinking. Now, if somebody doesn't take responsibility for the amount of thoughts they have and the flood of thoughts and discontinuity of thoughts and that whole tumultuous activity which goes on in the normal mind, then there's no way out of the morass, because that is basically what causes mental problems. So there has to be some kind of a sane relationship developed with one's own mind. Now that's a very big subject. We don't even have the tradition for it in this country. But maybe this kind of a discussion will establish that—the alternative is this: either people learn to control themselves or there will be a profession which will control them, because society is not going to stand for anything.

Farber: Well, with Kate, for example, it came to the sense of tolerating her own madness.

Leifer: Exactly. I happen to know Allen Ginsberg well. Maybe I shouldn't say this for publication, but there are people who can live with other people who maybe other people couldn't live with, tolerate their eccentricities and nurture them and let a lot of things go by, and not get all excited and learn to live a little closer to the edge. But if you're living with people who can't do that, you have to be dead and tight yourself.

Farber: Or dissimulate.

Leifer: Or dissimulate. Dissimulation is another whole skill.

Farber: And it's a worthwhile skill, I would think.

Leifer: Absolutely worthwhile skill. It's part of this learning how to stay out of psychiatric hands.

Farber: I remember—you know that guy, Bentov? He wrote a book on the brain as a holograph. He was interviewing some people in a mental hospital. He asked them why they were there. They said they heard voices. He said, "I hear voices, too." The patients said, "You hear voices? How come you're out there and I'm in here?" He says, "Because I shut up about it."

Leifer: Exactly. I had a call from Boston about somebody

who was in a mental hospital because she was
complaining about the Mafia being after her.
They asked for my help. I said, "Tell her to stop
saying the Mafia is after her." I took an hour to
explain how to get this message across to her.
Well, the person who gave her the message got it
across to her. She stopped talking about it, she
was out in two weeks. So let me summarize. The
so-called 'anti-psychotic' medicines and tranquilizers are basically anti-fear drugs in that they
interfere with the physiology of fear and thus give
a sensation of relief from fear to some people.
Other people, it just shuts down their motor energy systems to such a degree that they cannot
engage in this conduct.

Farber: That's what most of the people I interviewed said.

Leifer: The heavier psychotics tend to do that, they tend to
be more like PCP. Now, for humans PCP is so
toxic, you might say, that it causes mental manifestations, you might say psychedelic—I'm not
sure if they're psychedelic or deliriogenic. The
major tranquilizers are used to sort of paralyze
and immobilize humans so that they can be
brought under control. In order to get off that
kind of medication, a couple of things are necessary. One is gradual withdrawal, and then the
other is their taking over the function of the
drug, which means, if the purpose of the drug is
to reduce their anxiety, managing their own fear.
Their fear may be driving their behavior—when
people are afraid, they do things which, to other
people, may seem irrational, but to the person
who's afraid, it may just be a part of the fear. But
they then have to do something, if fear is the
problem, to manage their fear. And physical,
muscular relaxation, progressive muscular relaxation, is a very important tool in that. But also
some basic mind-stabilization exercises are important, in order to calm the mind, because a
very busy mind is prone to produce negative
emotions, especially fear. And so in people who
are experiencing fear you might say that to a

certain extent they're stimulating the fear state themselves. Or, to put it another way, they have the capacity, through acts of their own will, if they're designed well enough, to reduce their own mentation and reduce their own self-provocation and negative states, reduce their own fear.

Farber: Frequently the greatest fear is the thought that was planted in their mind by many, many authorities, 'If you go off this drug you're going to go crazy. Your illness will return.'

Leifer: Well, that's what you might call a secondary fear. There is a primary fear which precedes that, which was the reason they were put on the drug.

Farber: But that may no longer be there.

Leifer: That's right. Psychiatrists are not even interested in what that life issue is. They're only interested in bringing behavior under control, which is what's necessary in large mental hospitals in order to control the population. I worked at Pilgrim State Hospital in 1956, when Thorazine was first introduced. So I had an opportunity to observe what happened. The most visible change was that the attendants, who were very big and strong and carried large key rings with chains on them to both lock the doors and use as a weapon of self-defense, no longer had to carry those key chains. That's what the Thorazine did. Basically the Thorazine replaced the chains.

Farber: You, I imagine, advise people, if they ask for your advice, to get off Thorazine.

Leifer: Yes, I advise them to get off it as quickly as they can.

Farber: I think that makes you exceptional as a psychiatrist, wouldn't you say?

Leifer: I would say that I'm in a very small minority. I hardly know any others.

Farber: Well, Breggin, obviously.

Leifer: Breggin. I know one or two others, but it's a real handful, and to me that's a symptom of the official psychiatric suppression of thought. Because the official psychiatric position is that any deviation is contrary to American public health, just as deviation from the Communist Party line was considered contrary to the security of the state. The same rhetoric for repressing speech in Stalinist Russia is now being used by the American Psychiatric Association to prevent the kind of situation where people can pick, they can know which psychiatrist will tend to put you on drugs and which will tend to get you off. There is no such choice right now.

Farber: So a lot of people are going to have to do it without the support of a psychiatrist.

Leifer: A lot of them, that's right, will have to do it with a kind of indigenous foot-doctor of a new sort which arises from the masses in order to take care of this problem.

Farber: What about some of the obstacles, as Kate Millett found. People will interpret someone's behavior as pathological just because they know they're going off the drugs. What about obstacles like that?

Leifer: No, I don't think so, unless their behavior is becoming disturbing. And that's a fact that has to be faced, that what we're talking about here is a population of people who have disturbed some other people who are more powerful than they are, and these people have taken measures to bring them under control.

Farber: Kate describes behavior at times as eccentric, unusual, associations that one need not put a negative valuation on—but she also describes having a fight with her girlfriend, and her girlfriend getting irritated and saying, "Are you taking your Lithium?"

Leifer: Well, I read this in Kate's book. I would say that you cannot understand what happened to Kate there without knowing her girlfriend and what her girlfriend's contribution to that was. The full story is not being told there. There's some question as to whether, one, Kate was giving a full description of her behavior and, two, whether her friend, in particular, had a very low tolerance for deviance from her own standards of behavior and she just had the wrong friend at the moment, which could be quite possible also.

Farber: What about the more serious drugs like Thorazine? The neuroleptics? Are there any other obstacles? I mean, I presume that there are a series of obstacles relating to the way significant others are going to respond.

Leifer: When people go off the drugs their florid mentations may return.

Farber: Now Kate was obviously a hypermentative, imaginative person, who wouldn't want to lose those mentations, as was, you know, someone like James Joyce, for example.

Leifer: Exactly. But the task for these people is to learn some dissimulation, so that they're not losing what imaginative and creative aspect of that that they want to keep, and they're also not making a nuisance of themselves. So you have to learn some middle ground, where you appreciate the value of this and the beauty of this, and you acknowledge your excitement about it, but you also have to recognize that other people may not have the same enthusiasm for it as you do. You have to have the decorum and the self-control to not impose that on other people. If you can do that you don't need the medication.

Farber: Well of course, James Joyce or Kate Millett can sit down and write a book.

Leifer: Exactly. And there are lots of people who can't, and those are the people who get these medications.

Farber: So their imaginative possibilities are throttled because a negative valuation is placed upon those kind of unusual free associations in terms of thought processes.

Leifer: Or you might say, as a writer named Ed Powell would say, that it's a case of the imagination run wild. Or what he says is, intelligence run wild, which is quite true. You might say that psychosis is a matter of intelligence run wild. Powell recognizes that there is some positive value in it, some intelligence, some insight, some intuitions, some creative expressions, a lot of positive things, but it's run wild in the sense that it's experienced by other people as an assault. That may be a measure of their intolerance to it but could also be just, you know, quite obnoxious.

Farber: What's the difference between its running wild and its being obnoxious?

Leifer: The tolerance of the people around you. You could do it at a party, but maybe people don't want to hear it every day.

Farber: So it's a question of finding the right context?

Leifer: Exactly.

Farber: And it's a question of developing a tolerance for one's deviant thought processes.

Leifer: Developing a tolerance for it. But here's a Buddhist insight which is I think very helpful in this situation. A Buddhist lama observed that Americans have a tendency to want to be entertained and to have something intense happening every moment. It's what he calls an intolerance of boredom. And if that were reflected upon, it would I think be seen to be quite relevant to the problem of people who are getting medicated against their will. You know how I feel about the psychiatric establishment, so I don't need to preface this by saying I'm not defending them, but it's not just the psychiatric establishment that has to be viewed in this situation. It's also people who have no insight into, or no desire or ability to control their behavior and recognize the impact of their behavior on other people. Because if they did that, they would just simply not come to the attention of the authorities. Or if you did, you'd do it in some kind of a creative way which understood where the boundaries are. You know, our society is very busy drawing boundaries. Mapplethorpe is a boundary.

Farber: What's a boundary?

Leifer: Robert Mapplethorpe, that photographic display in

Cincinnati that's now being prosecuted, because certain people think it's obscene since it shows male genitals. There is a big issue now of the censorship of art. Well, what we're talking about is the censorship of people way, way inside that boundary; that is, people who are clearly disturbing somebody more powerful than they are, which is the issue in this photographic exhibit. This is a matter really of censorship; what we're talking about here is censorship and control.

Farber: And you're also talking about the kind of norm of sanity as a kind of colonialism, which is, you know, a Laingian theme and Kate Millett sounds it again. The idea that insane or unusual thought associations or dreamlike associations are to be negatively valued . . .

Leifer: There's that. There is the tendency on the part of society, of which psychiatry is a social agent, to control thought. But there's more than that. There is people's individual tolerance of being bothered by other people. That's at a very remote, non-intellectual, emotional level, non-ideological.

Farber: And isn't that also being bothered just by eccentricity?

Leifer: Yes, bothered just by eccentricity.

Farber: Which is perhaps another word for creativity?

Leifer: Yes, bothered by both.

Farber: So one of the things that's implied in persons learning to dissimulate is not interpreting their own unusual thought associations as symptoms of an illness.

Leifer: That's very important, not to buy that whole scheme at all. I know a lot of people who think their thoughts rush much too fast and too hard, and they're uncomfortable with them themselves, and would like to find some way to calm them down for their own sake. And there are other people whose mind is so busy that it spills over on other people, and they don't have any insight into that, and they first need to get insight into that, to see

how there is the potential for controlling one's
mind so that one doesn't become a nuisance to
other people.

Farber: And it's particularly important in light of the fact
that the psychiatric establishment has such power
that it ought not to have.

Leifer: That's one of the reasons for warning people against
the psychiatric establishment. What I say to people regularly is, 'Look, if you behave like that,
police will be coming after you. And they'll hand-
cuff you and put you in a police car and take you
to a place called the mental hospital. And you
ought to know that that may be the consequence
of your behavior, so that you can avoid that if
you want to. Think about that. This is leading
you in that direction.' Now that, in my observa-
tion, that kind of eye-opener brings a lot of people under control. They don't want that to
happen.

Farber: What about getting off Lithium?

Leifer: Getting off Lithium, now here's a problem. Let me
say a little bit about the antidepressants, getting
off the antidepressants. There are basically these
two main types of psychiatric drugs. One is an
anti-fear drug, we talked about that, the
phenothiamines and major and minor tranquilizers. The antidepressants basically are what you
might call psychic energizers. They do the opposite of what the tranquilizers do.

Farber: Yes, they mobilize the flight/fight reaction.

Leifer: They're basically speed, they're all basically speed.
Depression is not caused by some kind of a physical or genetic or neurophysiological deficit, but
rather it's caused by the loss of hope. Hope
moves us into the future, it's hope that motivates
us. Hope and motivation are two sides of the
same coin. So that when people for various
reasons—usually excessive and unrealistic hope
—find their hopes dashed, they lose hope and
that loss of hope bogs them down into a depression. The body then follows and they get dried up

and they need a motivator to get them going.

Farber: You could also call it a state of discouragement.

Leifer: You could call it a state of discouragement. And the antidepressants are basically courage drugs. So now this speed—incidentally, there are many people medicating themselves with speed voluntarily and illegally, and other people having it thrust upon them or sold to them for various reasons—but Prozac is basically speed. The antidepressants are basically speed. And a psychiatrist will jump on me about that and we could get into a technical discussion about it which I would enjoy. This may not be the place. The point is that when you're helping a person get off antidepressants you have to focus on their hope structures, that is, the way in which they perceive the future and their own motivations or reasons for living and acting and get them going again.

Farber: So you have to do various things to empower them.

Leifer: Empower them, help them to understand what depression is and help them to set up goals and projects which will move them into the future.

Farber: That was pretty clearly done with Aaron Beck. You know his work, cognitive therapy, and they've got the studies to prove that it works.

Leifer: Yes, it works for exactly that reason. People can have wrong ideas which discourage them, and then they can exchange those ideas to something more workable.

Farber: He also does behavioral things so they see themselves succeeding.

Leifer: Exactly. So that will work.

Farber: Now what about Lithium?

Leifer: Nobody understands how Lithium works. When I say what I think about it, it's just the way I think about it, not that I know how it works, because nobody knows that. But Lithium is one up on the Mendeleyev scale from sodium. And it's well known that sodium, the sodium pump, is what activates neural excitation, which is responsible

for nerve transmission. So it's not out of bounds
to speculate that Lithium, which is a more heavy
molecule, replaces some of the sodium and simply slows down the nervous system, which is exactly the way a lot of people experience it.

Farber: Even promoters of it say it 'turns down the dial of
life'.

Leifer: Exactly, exactly, it turns down the dial of life. Now
why is it turning down the dial of life? Because
certain people have gotten themselves so worked
up with energy of what you might call false hope
—you see, it's called bipolar disorder, and there's
a very good reason for calling it that, a bad reason and a good reason for calling it bipolar disorder. The bad reason is that there's a spurious
relationship between the psychiatric categories of
depression and mania. But the underlying reason
is that everybody goes through the process of
erecting hopes, having them dashed, going
through blue periods, getting yourself going again,
getting started up again. We're all on that kind of
a treadmill. Some people get on that in a more
extreme form. If their hopelessness is more extreme their mania can be more extreme, mania
being the state of excitation when your sense that
your going to achieve your outlandish hopes is at
its highest and you're filled with pride.

Farber: Often, people who've described this so-called manic
state have described it as an ecstatic state, the
same kinds of states that you'll find described in
the mystics at times.

Leifer: No, no. The Indian mystic is enstasy. It's totally
self-contained. There's a difference between ecstasy and enstasy.

Farber: Well, they have more control over it. They *learned* to
control it.

Leifer: You might say it's a state of enthusiasm. One, when
it's ecstatic it's expressed outwardly, the other
one gets expressed inwardly. The Indian mystic is
not out jumping around, spending money, walking down the street without any clothes on, pro-

voking policemen.

Farber: But Ramakrishna, he was in a state of ecstasy. He had to have someone to keep him from falling over.

Leifer: If you're defined as a guru and a special person who has assistants so that you don't need to carry money or figure out how to pay your taxes, then you can do that. If you have a support system, and people worship you, you can do that. But if you don't have a support system and people worshipping you, you're a pain in the ass.

Farber: Anyway, of course people, although they describe this as a pleasurable state, they get in trouble by running up high bills, and so forth.

Leifer: Exactly. That is how they get in trouble—spending money, having too much sex and provoking the police, or making too much noise and bothering their neighbors.

Farber: But it doesn't seem as if the answer should be to squash these states altogether.

Leifer: The psychiatric answer is to squash them, because it's the most ignorant approach to the situation and the most simple approach, just simply hit someone over the head. As opposed to try to understand them and try to talk with them and reason with them and give them techniques which would help them to be ecstatic without bothering other people. That's very difficult.

Farber: Can you think of a particular technique to be ecstatic without bothering people?

Leifer: Meditation.

Farber: Susan described dancing as a way of doing that. She's a professional dancer.

Leifer: Dance, art, yoga. Let me give you a definition of yoga given to me by my teacher, which is extremely relevant. Yoga means yoke, which comes from the metaphor of two oxen and a driver all yoked together. The oxen are yoked together but the driver is also connected to the yoked system. So it's a connectedness. Definition of yoga: how to

live in the outer world, how to live in the inner
world and to bridge the two. How to live with
your own mind and experience, how to live with
other people and how to bridge the two. Now to
me that's a perfect definition of psychotherapy.

Farber: What it should be, you mean.

Leifer: What it should be, and what's needed to get people
off these psychiatric drugs.

Farber: You would advise people to get off Lithium, also?

Leifer: I would advise them to get off all of those drugs.
Now the whole country is advising people to get
off marijuana, which is relatively harmless.

Farber: I know people who use marijuana to calm themselves
down and they find it very effective.

Leifer: There are a tremendous number of people medicating
themselves—if you want to call it a medicine,
I'm not sure I would even go that far—
administering substances to themselves to create
a state of mind that works for them. Others having it forced upon them. I would advise people to
get off all psychiatric drugs.

Farber: Would you say publicly that you think, for example, a
drug like marijuana has some benefits whereas
the psychiatric drugs don't?

Leifer: I would say first of all that marijuana is less harmful
and second of all, yes, I would go so far as to say
that it has some limited value. I don't want to
glamorize it; on the other hand I don't think it's
an evil substance.

Farber: And would you advise people also, if they're experiencing extreme anxiety, to take the least powerful
drug, for example to take a Valium rather than a
Thorazine?

Leifer: Absolutely. And preferentially start with something
very mild.

Farber: Like an herbal.

Leifer: Like an herbal, a valerian root or a glass of wine, or a
bath or an exercise bike, or relaxation exercises.
If those all don't work, take a small amount of
Valium while you're developing skills in these

other areas.

Farber: Yes, because this goes against the whole psychiatric ideology, because anything that makes a person feel good, like Valium or a glass of wine, they start screaming that the person is going to become addicted to it.

Leifer: Well, these drugs, if they bring you up to functioning like a social robot, they're called psychiatric medication. If they exceed that so that you feel good, they're called abuse.

Farber: So, basically getting off the Lithium is similar to the process you describe for getting off the neuroleptics?

Leifer: Sure. Although fear is not at the forefront in the so-called mania states. Yet I think mania states are fear-driven. But the fear is much more subtle and in the background and, you might say, dialectically being responded to while people who are being given neuroleptics are having an immediate experience of fear which is very tangible and present.

Farber: One woman I knew was having a number of visions that were quite ecstatic, but she hadn't slept, was afraid she couldn't take care of her kid, went over to her parents' house and then she became frightened, because they became frightened.

Leifer: Yes. If they hadn't become frightened it might have been quite possible . . . This is another thing that should be known: how to create a context for people who are fearful, which would help them to reduce the fear as opposed to accentuating it. Because if somebody comes in and they're very anxious, then that freaks people around them out, they take them up to the emergency room and they're thrust into that whole thing. They're at the peak of their fear and everyone's defining it as 'being taken care of', but it's the most frightening experience right at that point. I've always advocated putting people in a quiet room with quiet music, sip a little tea, don't say anything, lower the lights, a quiet room. A quiet room would work much better than any of the major tranquilizers. But actually, people coming in to get psychiatric care get provoked into more fear and anger.

Farber: When she was given the Thorazine her fear increased greatly, because her visions earlier, she said, were ecstatic, were pleasurable. But when they gave her the Thorazine, all of a sudden she felt as if her whole body were on fire.

Leifer: The neuroleptics cause a lot of very physical symptoms—plus you lose control of your mind. I mean, part of losing that hypermentation means that you can't understand what's happening to you. And you have to be sort of dummy-passive in order to get through it. If you're trying actively to figure out and take control you can get what's called a 'paradoxical response' to Thorazine and other major tranquilizers. In some individuals it increases their anxiety. To me that makes the most sense.

Farber: So you have helped people get off Lithium, for example?

Leifer: Yes, I have a whole group of people I helped get off of Lithium.

Farber: The kinds of techniques that you employ . . .

Leifer: Helping them increase control, recognize the effect of their behavior on other people, take measures to increase their own control of their behavior and speech, so that they don't provoke other people.

Farber: So they're able to experience altered states of consciousness and contain them without . . . they don't feel compelled to conform to what psychiatry says is the norm of sanity.

Leifer: No, you have to accept your status as an underground person *vis-à-vis* official psychiatry. It's very much like being Kierkegaard's underground person.

Farber: So you find that true with many people, they continue to have altered states of consciousness but they no longer bother other people?

Leifer: Exactly.

Farber: There's a phenomenon that Carl Jung called synchronicity—or mysterious, unusual coincidences—that I've experienced in my life quite frequently and I think people do experience that, and that might make them think they're going crazy, because it's not supposed to take place.

Leifer: Right. There are many things like that. Official reality is a very constricted view of the world, and so anybody who has not been robotized and tranquilized by social authority is going to have extraordinary states of consciousness which are neither comprehended nor condoned by official society. I think people are having those things, including transcendent states, all the time. They may be immanent states, they may not be transcendent. They just may be very immanent, poignant experiences of life which one doesn't have in the usual routine round of bureaucratic life. If you have a real-life experience it can make a very big impression on you.

Farber: So there are experiences that Maslow might call 'peak experiences' that would be positively valued in different spiritual traditions.

Leifer: They could be, although we want to be careful and not say that that's the rule. That's probably the exception. The rule is people who can't, who don't have enough self-discipline . . .

Farber: It could be both, couldn't it?

Leifer: Yes, it definitely could be both simultaneously.

Farber: So the key is developing self-discipline.

Leifer: To me that is very much the key, yes.

Farber: But we don't have . . .

Leifer: We don't have a tradition for that.

Farber: We don't have yogis to teach people, or shamans. There are a few, but most people end up in the hands of psychiatrists.

Leifer: A tremendous absence in our culture is the development of people who are skilled in self-control and can teach it to others.

PART THREE

In Revolt against the System

*Now you are flames, I'll teach
you how to burn.*

—JOHN KEATS *HYPERION*

CHAPTER THIRTEEN

To Break the Silence: George Ebert Speaks

George Ebert has been an activist in the mental patient liberation movement since 1978. George had the idea for the creation of Activists for Alternatives, which was founded by George, myself, and several others. He is director of the Mental Patients Alliance of Central New York, "a self-help and mutual advocacy organization" with state funding to operate a drop-in center. George's last incarceration in a psychiatric facility was in 1975. He felt his breakdown was a breakthrough. He believes he was guided by a higher power and he discovered that it was possible to reach a "higher level of existence".

George met his wife, Mary Ann, well before his institutionalization. Although not herself a 'survivor', Mary Ann is also an activist in the anti-psychiatry movement. The Eberts have two children who recently completed college.

George had been incarcerated three times. Each time he was told he had an incurable mental illness. "They would not let me out until I accepted that I was mentally ill, that I would be mentally ill forever and I would agree to take their drugs. . . . If I accepted what they were telling me about myself I couldn't accept myself." I asked him what were the factors that enabled him to reject their definition of him.

"Ah . . . it's not of my choosing."

Excerpt from George Ebert's Speech 'To Break the Silence'

A recent *Star Trek* rerun told a tale about a sub-class of people who were kept underground and in darkness. It was a story about their struggle to gain the same things that other people need—equality, kindness, and justice. A question about the treatment of these people was posed at a council meeting of the ruling class. The question was asked: "Are we so sure of our methods that we

187

never question what we do?" I hope to move you to question
what is being done to, and said about, real people in this real
time and real world.

I am thankful to be able to be present here today, for I am a
person who was silenced in the name of mental health. Silenced
because I could be certified as 'mentally ill'. I know what can
happen when a person questions authority, or challenges conformity or normality. I know that people are fragile and can be
broken. I am familiar with what the phenothiazine drugs do to a
person's ability to express one's self. I have no doubts that shock
treatment causes memory loss. I know what being caged, prod-
ded and provoked can do to one's spirit. I am speaking here
today from experience and about what can happen to a voiceless
people. I will address the barriers to justice.

One thing that happens is that other people categorize us. I do
not think it is accurate to identify people who are denied basic
human and civil rights, locked up in institutions, lied to, lied
about, and incapacitated as 'consumers' of mental health services. I do not think it is right to refer to people who have been
programmed into dependency, who exist under another's control
and authority, who have no voice, no choice, no opportunity for
informed decision-making and no representation as 'consumers'.
I feel that calling people who have been victimized by these
deprivations, and by isolation, with lobotomies, shock treatment, toxic drugs, behavior modification and experimentation
—that calling us 'the mentally ill'—adds insult to our injuries.

The 'no hope' diagnoses, the allegation that we are sick and
will always be sick, the claim that while our 'symptoms' may
possibly remit, by no means will we ever be well or whole, is a
curse. That idea that our psyches, our very souls are irreparably
diseased, is abuse.

This is not a mere semantic issue. What we call ourselves, how
we envision ourselves—and what others call us and how they see
us—can be crucial and is vital. In Nazi Germany mental
patients were called 'useless eaters' and 'people without value'.
Their extermination—initiated not by Hitler but by
psychiatrists—was termed 'euthanasia'. Now, however, the des-
ignated group, always a powerless and vulnerable people, is no
longer seen as useless, but as a financially valuable commodity.

The annual cost in dollars of the psychiatric system in New
York State in private and public monies exceeds five billion.
Imagine the differences, imagine the change, that could be
possible if that much money, if the woman- and man-power, the

time and energy expended, went into providing a humane habitat, human services and opportunity for equality—rather than psychiatric beds and total control over the lives of people who have special needs or present challenging problems.

The denial of the damage done to people by accepted treatment procedures is an abuse. The domination of psychiatric techniques over a multitude of methods of understanding, of serving, assisting, helping and healing people is an abuse. To hold the threat of further 'treatment' over the lives and minds of homeless people who have been so hurt and alienated that the streets offer more hope and refuge than the present system is an abuse.

Wolf Wolfensberger, professor at Syracuse University, has explained "how being devalued and rejected can jeopardize a person's life" and "how devalued people are being made dead in a systematic fashion". He submits that "it is time to cast off the web of disguise and deception that surrounds current genocidal practices, to proclaim the truth and oppose the forces of death-making".

See the people burned out by shock treatment and wiped out by psychosurgery. See the trembling, drooling, stumbling people who suffer the damage of tardive dyskinesia—those estimated 50 million victims of iatrogenic injury. See the reality of malignant neuroleptic syndrome and the thousands of deaths associated with that final solution for 'mental illness'. Recognize the devastation caused to humanity by psychiatric treatment.

Hear us. We are saying that individuals who have been psychiatrically labelled are full human beings. We are not defective, damaged, or mentally ill, although many of us have been physically harmed by psychiatric treatment. We are each a person. We are usually not what you call us or what you expect us to be. As long as the psychiatric state remains, as long as people are being tortured, oppressed, dehumanized, and denied ownership of their lives, we who have survived are obligated to struggle to break the silence.

CHAPTER FOURTEEN

From Victim to Revolutionary: An Interview with Leonard Frank

Frank: The story of the changes I went through began around 1959, when I was 27 years old.

Farber: You have indicated in your writings that there was some kind of spiritual transformation that took place in you at that time.

Frank: That's precisely the way I would put it, but the psychiatrists I encountered subsequently didn't see it that way. They saw what I was going through as a 'psychotic break'.

Farber: How did it all happen?

Frank: I had come out to San Francisco in 1959. I was born and brought up in Brooklyn, graduated from the Wharton School at the University of Pennsylvania, and after being drafted into the army for two years, I went to work as a real estate salesman in New York City. Following two years of fruitless activity in two different jobs, I moved to Florida to continue working in the real estate field. That didn't work out either, so I moved to San Francisco where after obtaining my real estate license I went to work for a downtown firm trying to sell or rent commercial properties. As you can see, I was relentless, or better still, a little slow in catching on to my basic unsuitability for that type of work.

[500]Leonard Frank was institutionalized for nine months in 1962. In 1974 he co-founded the Network Against Psychiatric Assault. He is the editor of *The History of Shock Treatment* (San Francisco, 1978) and the author of numerous articles. This interview was conducted in May 1991.

Incarceration and Torture

Farber: It sounds, however, as if you were pretty much a conventional sort of person in those days.

Frank: In retrospect, I was an extraordinarily conventional person—in my beliefs and in my lifestyle, right down the line. Like so many people with my background in that era, I was striving to 'make it'. In terms of my goals in life, I was a fifties 'yuppie'.

But after working for a few months in my new job, things began to change for me, more inside myself than externally. I was discovering a new world within myself, and the mundane world, comparatively speaking, seemed rather drab and uninteresting. I began reading non-fiction books and became very serious-minded. There was a big shift in my values and goals, and in my politics, too. I began recognizing my own prejudices and instances of injustice in the world about me. Now I began to see how the Golden Rule applied in business and politics: those who had the gold made the rules—and almost always to their own advantage.

At the same time, I continued working. After a few months, however, I became aware of the absurdity of my situation—the obvious clash between the direction of my emerging self and that of my old self—and lost interest in my job. Not surprisingly, I soon lost my job.

For a while I tried to find another one, but then I realized that being unemployed gave me a good opportunity to pursue my new interests in depth. So I started borrowing books from the library and buying used books. There was no pre-arranged course of study; it just seemed like one book led to another, one discovery to another. Soon I was busy rethinking everything; what was happening to me was that I was busy being born. As Dylan put it a few years later, "He not busy being born is busy dying". I came to see it that way too.

It was very exciting! The entire process seemed so natural. What guidance I needed came from within myself. I don't remember even seeking it; it was just there, somehow anticipating my needs before I experienced them. It was as though I was floating along on a river of enchantment and excitement, never knowing what to expect as I approached each bend, but seldom disappointed with what it turned out to be. Sure, I would occasionally bump into the debris of failings and regrets from my earlier life, but I was never bruised, and I just moved on undaunted and confident that I was doing the right thing. From books and from deep inside myself either intuitively or by way of dreams, new ideas—or at least ideas that were new to me—tumbled into my mind, but I never felt lost or confused. I simply mulled them over, selected out the best ones and began applying them in my own life.

In short order, I got away from being materialistic and became more idealistic and spiritual. I was thinking not only about my own well-being and that of my family, but also about how everyone could improve the quality of their lives. I soon gave up my meager job-seeking efforts altogether and stayed alone in my apartment absorbed in solitary study and reflection. This lasted for about two years.

During this period, my parents, who were then living in New York City, would visit me occasionally, and before long they became concerned about the person I was changing into. They preferred the person I had been, the person who I now saw as a caricature of the person I could be and was now becoming. So they tried to persuade me to change back into the person I had been. When their efforts failed, they concluded that there must be something seriously wrong with me and urged me to see a psychiatrist. I resisted. I said I was doing fine and didn't need a psychiatrist; I just wanted to pursue my studies and my new interests. It got to be a stalemate, and eventually they decided to force the psychiatrists on me. And the way that's done in our society is by commitment, which is a euphemism for psychiatric incarceration.

Farber: So you were actually committed against your will?

Frank: To say, "committed against your will" is redundant. When you're committed, that *is* against your will.

Farber: In their own terms, how could the psychiatrists justify doing this?

Frank: They said I was a 'psychotic', more specifically a 'paranoid schizophrenic', a term psychiatrists reserve for the most dangerous 'crazies', the serial murderers and people out of touch with 'reality'. My psychiatric records, which I obtained 12 years later in 1974, reported some of the 'symptoms' they used to justify locking me up and hanging that label on me. These included: not working, withdrawal, growing a beard, becoming a vegetarian, "bizarre behavior", "negativism", "strong beliefs", "piercing eyes", and "religious preoccupations". The medical examiner's initial report said that I was living the "life of a beatnik—to a certain extent".

Farber: That sounds almost comic except the consequences of it were so destructive.

Frank: Well, exactly. But even today, many people hearing about this would think that the very fact that I wasn't working, when I could have been if I wanted to, indicates that there was something very wrong with me. Once you stop working, or stop going to school, you're almost immediately going to raise suspicions about yourself. The underlying assumption is that there must be something wrong with you—either you're physically sick, which was ruled out in my case, or 'mentally sick'. If you're working and doing a reasonably decent job, not causing anyone a lot of trouble, not disrupting anything, you can believe and do —short of criminal activity—whatever you like no matter how outrageous.

In short, if you're earning a living—if you're

playing the game—almost anything goes; if
you're not, almost nothing does. People dropping
out of the game is very frightening to those re-
maining in it. People dropping out without sanc-
tions would set a bad example from the
standpoint of the stick-it-outs. If the dropouts
aren't punished, similarly inclined people might
be encouraged to follow their example, and soon
the game might have to be called for lack of
players—or at least the rules of the game might
have to be changed, and that's something people
generally don't like, especially if they happen to
be in the winning side at the time.

Farber: After you were committed, where were you sent?

Frank: First, to the psychiatric ward of Mount Zion Hospital
in San Francisco and after being held there a few
days to Napa State Hospital in Napa Valley,
about 75 miles northeast of San Francisco. I
spent a couple of months there and was then
transferred to Twin Pines Hospital, in Belmont, a
suburb community just south of San Francisco.

Twin Pines was a very expensive private sani-
tarium, with well-kept gardens, nicely-appointed
rooms, and good food (by hospital standards); it
was there that the atrocities were carried out—
the insulin coma and electroshock 'treatments'.
The lovely gardens and the rest were just
window-dressing for the dirty business that was
going on inside. Actually, I would have been better off at Napa State, where they *only* wanted to
electroshock me.

My parents' agent in making all the arrangements for my incarceration and 'treatment' was
Norman Reider, a nationally-known psychoanalyst, who had been trained at the Menninger
Clinic in the 1930s. His involvement illustrates
the close ties between psychiatry and psychoanalysis. Many psychoanalysts use or are associated
with private psychiatric hospitals where they
sometimes send their 'patients' or others who refuse to become their patients, which was the case
with me.

The public generally assumes, incorrectly so, that psychoanalysts just talk to people and don't, like other psychiatrists, force them into hospitals. But here was this prominent psychoanalyst, a 'talk therapist', not only locking me up but making arrangements for me to get shock 'treatment'. It's easy to see how psychoanalysis can serve as a cover for what's really going on in a 'therapy' situation. Since that time, I've always thought of psychoanalysis as the velvet glove on psychiatry's iron hand.

Farber: Yes, I think psychoanalysis provides the intellectual credibility that makes the whole psychiatric system saleable to people who consider themselves intellectuals. The analysts do their labelling and 'talk cure' . . .

Frank: But they don't usually do the shocking; they only make the arrangements for the recalcitrant ones to be shocked. Reider, when he was at the Menninger Clinic worked with psychiatrists who used Metrazol, an early but particularly harsh form of shock, during which the subject was mostly conscious. Psychoanalysts and psychiatrists may clash publicly on minor issues, but they're cut from the same cloth: practically all of them use lock-ups, psychiatric drugs, and electroshock, or are at least complicit in these practices because they don't protest against them.

Farber: How long were you locked up?

Frank: All told, I was institutionalized for about nine months: the last seven at Twin Pines, where for three of those months I was forced to undergo combined insulin-electroshock, a total of 85 shock 'treatments'—50 insulin comas and 35 electroshocks. There was a court order which authorized it. My father had signed the consent form.

These so-called treatments literally wiped out all my memory for the two-year period preceding the last procedure. The period of self-conversion, except for its early stages, was erased from my mind in a brainwashing procedure tyrants from

all ages would have envied. There were also big
gaps in my memory covering earlier life experiences. My memory had been so devastated by the
shocking that afterwards I was surprised to find
out that John F. Kennedy was President of the
United States, although he had been elected two
and a half years earlier. Soon after the shocking
ended, I realized that my high-school and college
were all but gone; educationally, I was at about
the eighth-grade level. For the most part, the
memories never came back spontaneously. Some
few did, but almost all of what I know from the
two-year period preceding the last shock and
from much of my earlier life other people had to
tell me about.

Escape

Farber: How did you finally get out?

Frank: Basically, the way I did it was to compromise, to play
their game as I thought they wanted me to play
it. I just surrendered, at least outwardly. But I
never gave up my beliefs, or what remained of
them in my mind; I merely suspended my practicing them for the duration of my stay at Twin
Pines. I shaved voluntarily, ate some non-
vegetarian foods like clam chowder and eggs, was
somewhat sociable, and smiled 'appropriately' at
my jailers. In his correspondence to my father at
that time Robert E. James, the psychiatrist who
administered most of the shocks to me, noted
these changes as signs of improvement.

After 85 shocks I was on the road to 'recovery'. Had I been part of a clinical study on combined insulin-electroshock, I would have been
reported as one of the 'successful' cases. I had
been reduced—more or less—to the person the
evaluating psychiatrist thought I had been before
I had started transforming myself. That was their
standard of 'success'.

I was held at Twin Pines for about a month

after the shocking. My memory for this period is spotty. There was T.V. watching, 'occupational therapy', a few brief interviews with psychiatrist James, pills and mouth checks, a bowling outing, a dental appointment or two, but there was no further brutalization or even harassment. The worst of it was over with the last insulin coma, at least as far as I know from direct memory. The strongest memory I have from the entire period was coming out of the last coma, which also happened to be the only memory I have about any of the shocks. Returning to consciousness that last time was the worst, most painful experience of my life. The only reason why it stuck in my memory was that there were no succeeding shocks to blot it out.

Farber: Were you supposedly unconscious during most of these procedures? Were they using anesthetics in those days?

Frank: I don't know about that from my own experience. From what I've read about insulin coma in the professional literature, there is, leading up to a one-hour period of coma—and unconsciousness—a four- or five-hour period, during which the subject is mostly conscious, sweats and salivates profusely, experiences 'hunger excitement' (a psychiatric euphemism for intense hunger pain manifested by weeping and screaming), and often goes into convulsions.

These are the inevitable consequences of blood-sugar-depletion from the insulin which is injected at the beginning of the procedure early in the morning. An insulin coma is not unlike a 'diabetic coma', to which diabetics are subject. The difference is that in diabetes the coma happens naturally, or spontaneously, and is treated by physicians as a life-threatening emergency, while psychiatrists induce the coma artificially and regard it as a 'treatment'.

Farber: By what logic could they justify such an obscenity?

Frank: Well, the psychiatrists have provided themselves with quite a few theories about this over the years.

The one that stands out in my mind from all those that I've read about was formulated by Manfred Sakel, the Austrian psychiatrist who himself introduced the insulin-coma procedure as a treatment for 'schizophrenia' in the early 1930s. He believed the problem with schizophrenics was that their brains were dysfunctional and that with insulin he could literally 'kill' off the dysfunctional brain cells and thus liberate the normal ones. Even if you accept his assumption that schizophrenia is a brain disease, you have to go way beyond the imagination, let alone the scientific evidence, to accept his claim that with insulin comas he could selectively destroy the diseased brain cells.

Nevertheless, I've seen this theory mentioned with approval, or at least without criticism, a number of times in the psychiatric literature. The absence from professional writings of critical reporting and analysis concerning insulin coma was, I believe, an important factor in the relatively long life, about 25 years, the procedure had as a primary treatment for schizophrenia. A San Francisco psychiatrist, for example, once told me that while he was in training at the Menninger Clinic in the early 1950s it was decided to close the insulin ward because patients on the ward had been "dying off like flies". Had the Clinic's world-famous *Menninger Bulletin* carried an article reporting the facts surrounding the closing of this ward, the profession might have abandoned insulin coma in the mid-1950s, ten years earlier than it actually did.

But psychiatric journals, which most people regard as scientific, simply don't publish articles detrimental to the interests of their subscribers or advertisers. What these journals publish is the profession's conventional wisdom, a mess of errors and lies set forth authoritatively in pseudomedical language. Between the covers of these journals psychiatrists lie to themselves and each other. Then later, seeing their own lies in print, they believe them.

With regard to insulin coma, right from the start, published reports were virtually unanimous in support—remarkable results for previously 'hopeless cases', high recovery rates, grateful families, minimal risks, and on and on. You rarely get from them more than a hint of the ordeal subjects experienced during the procedure, especially its pre-coma phase. To understand what that was like, you have to read between the lines of what the psychiatrists wrote. For example, in one article an insulin-coma psychiatrist advised against allowing new insulin 'patients' to see all at once the sight of other patients in the different stages of the procedure—"a sight which is not very pleasant to an unaccustomed eye". I don't remember ever having seen such a sight, but I have the vivid recollection of hearing, after my own series had been completed, the screams of someone else who was undergoing combined insulin-electroshock in another area of the building where I was: they were like the screams you would expect to hear coming from a torture chamber.

I wanted to say something further about my amnesia from the combined insulin-electroshock, which, I believe, was the standard technique— insulin by itself was infrequently used. One of the memories the procedure destroyed was that I had begun growing a beard shortly before being committed. I know this from a mugshot that had been taken of me soon after being committed—it became a part of my psychiatric records. In addition, there was constant reference to the beard in the records: from the start the psychiatrists wanted me to shave it off, but I had refused. Eventually, while I was in an insulin coma and obviously unable to resist, the psychiatrists had my beard removed. According to the records, they justified this measure as a "therapeutic device" and besides, one of them noted, I could always grow another beard. This was done to me, according to psychiatrist James, in spite of the fact that I had attached "a great deal of religious significance to the beard".

Farber: That's almost like a symbolic castration.

Frank: Perhaps, and it was also a way of asserting their
power over me. It was like their saying to me,
You cannot be who you want to be: you will be
who *we* want you to be—and there's not a damn
thing you can do about it! It was still another
gross violation of my human rights. That shaving
off my beard was done in the name of 'therapy'
gave it legitimacy. Think about it: in our society,
therapeutic necessity, as determined by psychiatrists, has precedence over religious liberty.

   The Nazis also cut off beards. Do you ever
remember seeing the photograph of a bearded
concentration-camp inmate? In the Middle East,
going back many centuries, beard-shaving was
employed to humiliate individuals who society
wanted to punish, but in the latter half of the
twentieth century, in the land of Washington, Jef-
ferson, and Lincoln, the same method was used
supposedly to assist in the process of restoring an
individual to 'sanity'. Some might argue that this
trampling of my religious freedom which happened almost 30 years ago couldn't happen today.
While I can't cite any specific instances, I know it
certainly could happen today. This is born out by
a psychiatric resident's letter published two years
ago in *Dendron* which reported a sign near the
inpatient ward at the Mental Health Center in
Albuquerque which read, "Patients' Rights: Patients have the right to religious freedom unless
clinically contraindicated".

Farber: It must have been something to be in such a high
state of consciousness and making all these discoveries, and then to be plunged into this pit of
Hell.

Frank: I saw it that way too, and did so almost immediately
after coming out of that last coma. Despite the
disorientation—I didn't know where I was or
even what year it was—I knew that I had been
badly damaged and was in a desperate situation,
with my life hanging in the balance. In a little

while, I began picking up the bits and pieces of memory from my past life. The most recent memories I could recall were from the beginning stages of my conversion period.

I remembered reading the Bible and having become interested in spiritual matters. Then at Twin Pines, when the shocking was over, I was fortunate in being able to get hold of a Bible, a shortened, pocket-sized version published for GIs during World War II. I read it with staff consent —nothing I did at Twin Pines was without it— and was encouraged to find that at least some parts were still familiar to me. Even more important, the Bible was still able to inspire me with its message of hope. So I began retracing my steps.

In June of 1963 I was released from Twin Pines—the psychiatrists were apparently convinced that I would be a 'good boy', get a job, and take their pills. I don't know what kind they were, but while there they had tried me out briefly on Prolixin, which had then just been introduced. Although I don't remember this at all, my psychiatric records indicate that I had a terrible reaction to this drug and they switched me to another kind of . . .

Farber: Neuroleptic.

Frank: You say, "neuroleptic," but some people call the neuroleptics (like Prolixin, Haldol, and Thorazine), neuro*toxics*. Toxic means poisonous, which is what these drugs are. They not only weaken you, cloud your mind and make you feel awful when you take them, but when used for long periods of time, they can have devastating effects on your brain. Studies show the neurotoxics cause tardive dyskinesia, an often permanently disfiguring muscular disorder in 20–65 percent of longer-term users. This condition is almost invariably accompanied by tardive dementia, a kind of dementia which severely hinders your ability to think and feel. An estimated three million people in the United States alone take these drugs on a regular basis. Referring to tardive dyskinesia, my friend, psychiatrist Peter Breggin has written, "Psychiatry has unleashed an epidemic of neurologic disease on the world . . .[which is] among the worst medically-induced disasters in history."

Farber: And, of course, the psychiatric system today won't let people get off these drugs easily. There's a tremendous amount of pressure on people labelled 'mentally ill' to stay on them indefinitely, which sometimes means for the rest of their lives.

Frank: That's something I've made a point of in the past. Not only is there pressure, but consent, when it is obtained, is often based on misinformation about drug risks. I also believe that the neurotoxics, when heavily used, can be as harmful as electroshock, just as a large number of electroshocks can be as damaging as a lobotomy. These three psychiatric 'treatments'—drugs, electroshock, and psychosurgery (yes, brain operations are still being used to cure 'mental illness')—are at different points along the same continuum: each in varying degrees impairs mental functioning by irreparably damaging the brain.

Farber: How do you explain the reliance on drugs in our society?

Frank: I think it's obvious that we live in a drug-oriented culture. Everyone is looking for the easy solution, which in our culture gets translated into the quick fix. If it's not one kind of drug, it's another that will do the job. But mind- or mood-altering drugs offer no genuine solutions to the real problems most people face. What they offer is escape from them, and that of a very temporary sort. That applies to street drugs, alcohol, and over-the-counter drugs—as well as psychiatric drugs.

Moreover, the price that drug-users must pay for this momentary relief from the pressures and pains of living can be fearsome, for every hit entails the risk of a certain amount of brain-cell destruction. Any drug strong enough to affect your thinking or your mood is probably strong enough to damage your brain, however slightly. Some might argue that the brain has many billions of cells and it can afford to lose a few here and there on occasion, especially when one is miserable or looking for a kick.

Users should also know that the brain-damaging effects of these drugs are cumulative and can be disastrous in the long run. To some degree at least the various forms of dementia now showing up in younger and younger age groups and the senility afflicting older people in dispro-portionately larger numbers may be the conse-quence of the legal, as well as illegal, mind-altering drug craze that has been sweeping the country for the last 40 years. And isn't it ironic that psychiatrists, through their prescribing prac-tices, are helping to create the very conditions society usually calls upon them to treat?

Another thing to consider in connection with drugs is that the distress drug-users are trying to escape from can be used as a tool for their own growth and development. Someone once said, "Discontent is the parent of progress". Pain, dis-comfort, anxiety, and unhappiness are signals that there are problems in our lives that need attention. Left unanesthetized, these signals com-pel us to find or create solutions for our prob-lems. If anesthetized, they no longer act as incentives, so we do nothing and our problems are likely to worsen.

Farber: How long did it take you before you regained your equilibrium after having been through this horrif-ic experience?

Frank: After being released from the institution I moved into an apartment in San Francisco, where I still live. There I holed myself up for five or six years, re-reading at first the books I had read during the two-year period preceding the shocks. But just remembering which books they were was a prob-lem. All I had to go on were vague memory traces of what I had been reading: all the papers and books I had accumulated during that period had been lost. But bit by bit I re-acquired some of the knowledge that I had lost as a result of having been shocked and also went on to acquire new knowledge. I also had to relearn much of the English language; I had forgotten the meaning of many once-familiar words and had difficulty using correctly the words I still understood.

Farber: Because of the brain injury?

Frank: Yes. In addition, where there is a global amnesia, such as I had, there's going to be a learning disability. So it was very difficult, and it still is very difficult, for me to learn things. Memory and learning work together, and if your memory is impaired, your ability to learn is likely to be impaired to the same degree. That's been a struggle. It took me about six years of concentrated reading and study to get back to what I believe was my previous level of learning. In raw intellectual ability, I don't think I ever got back to my previous level. But in neither of these two matters can I speak with any assuredness. It's hard for me to estimate what my losses in this area were, just as it would be hard for anyone to know what they've lost when they can't remember what they had.

    Though my memory is still poor, I can usually hold onto things that are important to me. But I have to work at it. Constant mental activity, including study, enables me to make the most of the intellectual resources I still have. I also get a lot of help from 'crutches', like scratch-sheets and notebooks, and, in recent years, a computer. I'm forever making notes to myself of words, facts, and ideas which interest me. Later, I review them for possible inclusion in one of my notebooks or in the computer where I keep this information sorted out in categories by subject and/or source.

Religious and Intellectual Influences

Farber: Before continuing with your life story after being released from Twin Pines, I would like to go back to what you have called your "conversion period", particularly the books that influenced you at that time.

Frank: One such book was Mohandas Gandhi's autobiography. That book, perhaps more than any other, played the key role in changing my outlook. It marked the beginning of my interest in spiritual matters.

Farber: Before that, had you been religious in any sense?

Frank: No, although I had been raised as a Jew and had taken a few classes in my synagogue's Hebrew school, I wasn't at all interested in religion before moving to San Francisco. My family belonged to a Conservative synagogue, and though we attended services on the High Holy Days, we were far from being 'religious', observant Jews. Very little of Judaism rubbed off on me during my early years, at least consciously.

Farber: What was there about Gandhi that impressed you?

Frank: His sincerity, his values, his entire approach to life. It was completely new to me. His *Autobiography* is about his "experiments with truth", which is its subtitle. In it he recounts the progress of his own inner development and how this progress affected the course of his personal, professional and political life. With Gandhi, the inner and the outer worlds were never worlds apart; they interacted with and complemented each other. And, of course, much of the book concerned the principles and practice of nonviolence, with which I was unfamiliar till then.

The book also introduced me to vegetarianism. Like most Indians, Gandhi had been brought up as a vegetarian, but as a youngster had eaten meat on several occasions. He described one such break with the family tradition. He and a friend would secretly go off by themselves after school to eat goat's meat. They thought they could acquire the strength of the English, who at the time dominated India both culturally and politically, by imitating their meat-eating ways. Afterwards,

Gandhi began to have some moral qualms about this practice, but what really made him feel guilty and convinced him to give up meat-eating altogether was a dream he had following one of these escapades. In this dream, he heard the bleating of a goat coming from his own stomach.

That really struck home to me for it was about this time that I had begun paying attention to my own dreams, particularly their moral content. Gandhi's dream, as I then saw it, was as important to me as it had been for him. It sensitized me to the fact that animals had feelings and could suffer. I concluded that meat-eating was cruel and that I had no right to impose suffering on other creatures either *directly* by killing them myself or *indirectly* by having others kill them to satisfy my appetite for their flesh in return for money. It occurred to me that we can't avoid harming ourselves when we harm other beings, whether human or animal. Meat-eating was an excellent example of how this principle played out in real life. Gandhi, in his *Autobiography* and other writings, explained how meat-eating, because it was inherently cruel to animals and morally wrong, affected the wrongdoers by causing them to become sick and cutting short their lives.

So I became a vegetarian, and later a vegan, which means that I don't eat or use any animal products. I also became interested in nonviolence and began reading other writings by Gandhi on the subject. I soon decided that nonviolence was a valid approach to political problem-solving and became myself a nonviolent person. Instead of meeting force with force, you meet force with gentleness and active, nonviolent resistance. Because Gandhi's nonviolence was based on moral and spiritual values, I now turned my attention to the religious writings that he said had influenced him. Among the writings he cited were the *Bhagavad Gita,* the New Testament (especially the Sermon on the Mount), and Henry David Thoreau's 'Essay on Civil Disobedience'.

Farber: Wasn't it particularly the Sermon on the Mount that he was moved by?

Frank: Perhaps, but it was the thrust of the New Testament, as I was eventually to find out, that whole approach to dealing with problems with kindness and love, that I came to see as a practical alternative to the violence and counterviolence that was tearing our world apart. Before reading the New Testament, however, I read the Old Testament. I had thought to myself, well, here I am, a Jew, who has never even read the Old Testament, on which Jesus, the central figure of the New Testament, had based many of his ideas, and that I'd be able to understand his ideas better if I read the two books in their natural sequence. So I read the Old Testament first.

Farber: The whole Old Testament?

Frank: I'm not saying I read it word for word. I skip-read parts of it. For example, I didn't care much about the 'begats'—'Joseph begat Ham who begat Shem', and suchlike. What got me involved was the spirit of the book—it spoke to my heart, because my heart was ready for it. I was changing inwardly, and the Old Testament addressed the issues that were now becoming important to me. And what impressed me most were the experiences and teachings of the prophets.

Farber: Just looking at you—I mean, with your flowing beard, you look like an Old Testament prophet. Those pictures I've seen of you . . .

Frank: Well, that's been said. But I want to go on. In my heart I feel that the teachings of the prophets are valid for myself and also for our time, perhaps even more so than when they were first spoken. Until reaching that conclusion after my first reading of the Old Testament when I was about 28, I would have laughed in the face of anyone who suggested that I would come to believe something like that.

 The prophets' message was both personal and social. They were obviously very concerned about injustice. They believed that individuals could

not have a good relationship with God so long as
they misconducted their lives, that the highest
point of spiritual awareness could not be
achieved without righteous deeds.

They called upon their people to end their
violence, and their exploitation of one another.
The people heard the message but didn't heed it,
so one disaster after another fell upon them, even
up to our own time. And now the prophetic message is applicable not just to a people but to all
humanity. And, in my view, if it isn't heeded,
there will be a disaster of such magnitude that
Auschwitz, by comparison, would seem no more
tragic than stubbing your toe.

Farber: Which prophets are you referring to?

Frank: Basically, they all carried the same message. But it
was Isaiah who I found to be most inspiring. His
message—actually there were three authors of the
Book of Isaiah—was not merely beautiful poetry;
it was the highest understanding of God's ways
up to that point in human history. What Isaiah
said was more than something out of his imagination; it came from on high and was based on
dreams, visions, revelations, and mystical
encounters—experiences common to all humanity. Isaiah differed from most of the rest of us in
knowing from whence they came and in ascribing
great importance to them. But the raw material
of spiritual experience was no more available to
Isaiah than it was to anyone else living in his
time, or for that matter to anyone living today.

Farber: Can you put Isaiah's message in one or two sen-
tences?

Frank: I've already spoken about my understanding of the
prophetic message. Isaiah's was not that much
different from that of the other prophets. He
stressed the importance of justice and righteousness as the ways to redemption and self-realization, and gave an extraordinary preview of the
transitional period possibly leading into a new
age for humanity and, indeed, for all the earth's
creatures, a time of universal peace when

swords will be beaten into plowshares—but only after hearts of stone are changed into hearts of flesh.

Central to his vision, which he was not the only prophet to speak of, was the idea of a holy people. But I would extend this concept to the entire species. We human beings are a *holy species* destined to be given the chance to lead the entire Earthly creation in its transformation. If we so choose, we can become God's partners in fulfilling His dream.

Involved here is not just one people but all peoples, the whole human race. Among all of the Earth's creatures—I remember reading somewhere that there are 30 to 40 million species of life on Earth—we can play the pivotal role in transforming this little neck of the galactic woods, what has been for so many 'a vale of tears', into an Earthly paradise. To me, this is more than a *re*volutionary idea—it's an *e*volutionary idea.

Farber: These are certainly unorthodox ideas. How did the psychiatrists respond to them?

Frank: I don't recall ever having discussed these ideas with them. I don't even remember having had these specific ideas at that time although I think I was moving in that direction. For some people, beliefs such as these seem to be part and parcel of the conversion experience; for psychiatrists, they're the sure indicators of madness. I've been thinking about this subject lately, and the role psychiatry plays in suppressing unorthodox views, especially in the area of human spirituality. That's what I believe happened in my own case: I was going through a spiritual renewal, of which these or similar views were an accompaniment. It was a reborning process, which psychiatry tried to abort. The renewal process I experienced was a life-enhancing boon. It turned destructive only after psychiatry intervened with its so-called treatments. Had the process been allowed to run its course, who can say for sure what would have happened? My own opinion is that the 'treatments' set me back, to use the psychiatric term, 'regressed' me to an earlier phase of my development; without them, I would have been further along on the path than I am now.

Farber: That's the story of a number of people who I interviewed for this book.

Frank: That doesn't surprise me. But to back up a bit, it's hard to talk about one's own spiritual experience in a plausible way. People who haven't had that kind of experience find it extremely difficult to understand. What is more, I can't prove or demonstrate that what was happening to me inwardly was beneficial, or even that it was happening to me at all. It's strictly a matter of belief and interpretation. The problem of communication is made all the more difficult because in our scientific age, spirituality, which cannot be verified by the scientific method, doesn't have much credibility. With psychiatrists, who regard themselves (and are regarded by most people) as leaders in the field of human science, spirituality has even less credibility.

This phase of human evolutionary development is marked by its partial knowledge which is mistaken for being complete. In the next evolutionary phase this will become clear to us. In my opinion the transition period leading into this phase is about to begin. We stand at the dawn not just of a new historical era but of the next and culminating phase of human evolution; history and evolution are about to fuse. Unlike past evolutionary transitions which were forced and unconscious, the next one will be voluntary, involving a conscious, informed choice, by every member of the species.

And here I will again refer back to the Old Testament, this time to the occasion when Moses confronted his people with an either/or choice, "I have set before you life and death, the blessing and the curse, therefore choose life." He was anticipating the Day of Judgment, which may be seen as more like the Day of Choice. If we make the right choice, we can move ourselves and our species up the evolutionary scale, which would lead, in religious terms, to the establishment of the Kingdom of Heaven on Earth. The wrong choice would result in a calamity of barely imaginable proportions, a kingdom of Hell on Earth.

Because of our technological knowledge, we have the ability to make it go either way. With the proliferation of nuclear bombs and nuclear plants, we have the destructive power to make the earth a Hell. With television, radio, and satellite communication, everyone on Earth can almost simultaneously receive the message of the coming Kingdom of Heaven and learn what is required of them to bring it about. What I am getting at here is personal and social change through the spiritual conversion or evolutionary transformation of the entire species.

The British historian Arnold Toynbee influenced my thinking about such possibilities and the function served by civilization in this process. He used the chariot as a metaphor. The various civilizations were the wheels that carried the chariot forward. The chariot symbolized religion. He saw civilization as the means whereby religion was advanced. All civilizations went through periods of birth, growth, stagnation, and decline. During the decline phase, which is characterized by widespread institutional breakdowns, disillusionment, and loss of faith, they become receptive to new, and higher, religions.

Toynbee believed Western civilization in our age is analogous to the Roman Empire during its decline phase, and just as the roads, sea-travel, mail service, and so forth, developed by the Romans paved the way for the spread of Christianity throughout the Mediterranean World, so advances in communication and transportation pioneered in the Western World have set the stage for the conversion of all humanity to a higher religion. As the Romans adopted Christianity,

more or less out of desperation and in order
to survive, so world civilization today, with
the added fear of nuclear annihilation, is ripe
for adopting a new religion—in order to save
itself.

In my opinion, Toynbee, with this formulation,
hit upon a basic, recurring theme in human history.

In 1945, soon after atom bombs destroyed two
Japanese cities, killing more than 200,000 people,
Albert Einstein, without referring to Toynbee,
lent his support to at least one component of his
theory. In an interview, Einstein said, "For the
present [atomic energy] is a menace. Perhaps it is
as well that it should be. It may intimidate the
human race into bringing order into its international affairs, which without the pressure of fear,
it would not do."

Farber: Toynbee's theory reminds me of the twelfth-century
Christian mystic named Joachim of Fiore, who
prophesied that there was going to be in the future a new revelation which he called the "Age of
the Spirit". The Age of the Father from the Old
Testament and the Age of the Son from the New
Testament would be superceded by the Age of
the Spirit in the coming age. Merezhkovsky, a
Russian Christian mystic, said the Holy Spirit is
feminine. The Aramaic word for spirit is *ruach*
and its gender is feminine. He said that neither
the Father nor the Son had saved the world,
but that one day the Holy Spirit, the Mother,
would.

Frank: Some have regarded Judaism as a Father religion and
Christianity as a Son religion. Perhaps, the new
religion will be neither a Father nor a Son nor a
Mother religion—but a Brother/Sister religion.

Farber: By the way, are you familiar with Abraham Heschel's
work?

Frank: Yes, very much so. As a matter of fact, the book I'm
working on right now, which is a book of quota-
tions, includes many of his teachings culled from
the six or seven books of his that I've read.

Farber: He's a beautiful writer and very much in the Prophetic tradition, I would think.

Frank: No question about it! Interestingly enough, one of his books is entitled *The Prophets,* and it's well worth reading. I wanted to get back to Jesus for a moment. I was greatly impressed with his dedication, his belief in a higher purpose to life than was generally perceived, and his willingness to serve God regardless of personal consequences. I soon came to see Gandhi and Jesus as parallel figures in a way. The two men had mixed religion and politics which I had always seen, until my awakening, as separate entities.

Of course, as I said before, I didn't limit my reading to Jesus and Gandhi. Until moving to San Francisco I had never been much of a reader. As a student, my reading was restricted to class assignments, and I read only what was necessary to obtain a passing grade. In my twenties, I had done some fiction reading, but little in the way of non-fiction reading other that what was related to my business career.

Now I really pushed ahead. Gandhi had mentioned Thoreau. His 'Essay on Civil Disobedience' was for me, as it had been for Gandhi, an eye-opener. Here was the clear expression of some of the most important principles of nonviolence. Later I found out that Thoreau himself had actually put this creed into practice: He once went to jail briefly becuase of his principled refusal to pay a war tax. It was during the Mexican War in the late 1840s. He saw it as an unjust war and refused to co-operate with the government in paying for its cost. Here was good example of nonviolence in action.

I also read some of Tolstoy's writings, because Gandhi had mentioned him in his *Autobiography.* Gandhi had corresponded with Tolstoy in the early 1900s and was much influenced by him, especially with the idea of setting up small, mostly independent, nonviolent communities. Gandhi was then living in South Africa, where he established the first of a number of such communities, calling it Tolstoy Farm. After reading Tolstoy, I went on to read about Abraham Lincoln, another God-centered individual.

Farber: I didn't know that.

Frank: Not many people do. The Lincoln most people know comes from the standard history texts which portray him as a political figure. But when I looked into the heart of the man as evidenced by his own writings, I discovered that his political life was but an extension of the spiritual journey upon which he had embarked.

Farber: You know, I have been inspired by the same archetype. The person who had the most influence on my spiritual and intellectual development was probably Aurobindi Ghose. He was a contemporary of Gandhi's and died in 1950. He was very active in the Indian Nationalist Movement. It was when he was imprisoned by the British that he began to have mystical experiences. I think during the first such experience he saw every prisoner as a manifestation of Krishna (or God). Eventually he left the Nationalist Movement and became a yogi. Nevertheless, he continued to support the Movement, believing that there was no dichotomy between spiritual and worldly pursuits. On the contrary, Indian philosophy, in his view, had made a mistake—perhaps a necessary mistake but one that had to be transcended—in positing Nirvana (or Heaven) apart from this material world. The whole emphasis of his spirituality was on the transformation of this world.

Frank: Very interesting! I think that's one of the reasons we—you and I—connected. It's because our beliefs on this crucial point are so similar. But I wanted to finish up a few thoughts I had about Lincoln. As with Jesus and Gandhi, he believed he was being guided by God and that he was serving His will. The Civil War, as Lincoln understood it, was a means to some purpose that was beyond the consciousness of the participants, a means to some purpose that would be fulfilled in time, if not in his own time: in his words, "some wise purpose . . . mysterious and unknown to us." Something was being worked out on a higher level, which not even he could quite grasp, and the suffering and bloodshed of that terrible war, which he himself felt so deeply, was not in vain. I came to see that what Lincoln believed about the Civil War was no less true of the even crueler wars that have taken place during the twentieth century. It's almost inhuman to understand, let alone justify, something like the Holocaust or the nuclear bombing of Hiroshima and Nagasaki in this light. Still, I believe they serve some 'wise purpose' not yet known to us.

Dreams and Visions

Farber: One could, perhaps, say that evil must come to the surface before it can be overcome or transcended.

Frank: That's one way of looking at it. Maybe we're in a phase of human development where we have to go through the very worst in order to become the very best. In order to fulfill our potential as human beings, we have to understand our capacity for evil, too. Something John Lennon once said, in my opinion, applies well to the human condition: "We're all Christ; we're all Hitler." Accepting this idea about ourselves is in my view, if not the beginning of wisdom, close to it.

It's all within ourselves, the potential for holiness as well as for evil. The way we think and act shapes our character and determines the course of our lives. As the French philosopher Henri Bergson once wrote, "The world is a machine for making gods." Of course, the age-old question is how we become gods. That entails a search within ourselves for the light that will reveal the path to self-realization, which in its highest expression is God-realization. At the end of the path is oneness with God; we become at one with God, there is atonement, or at-one-ment. The path is open to everyone because God is in everyone.

This concept is a fusion of eastern and western belief and might be called pantheistic monotheism: God is One; God is all—God is One in all. All the differences which divide human beings from one another are transcended in the knowledge of our oneness with God.

Some have called travelling this path the 'inner journey', but it's really one, all-encompassing journey with an inner and outer aspect. One phase is primarily 'inner,' the other, primarily 'outer'. Toynbee spoke of this journey in terms of "withdrawal and return". During withdrawal, there is a reaching into the depths of oneself, acknowledging one's deficiencies, guilts, inferiorities, and fears. It requires courage and faith—and, more important, grace—to go through this garbage, but it's absolutely essential in order for transformation to take place.

Metaphorically speaking, there's no way to gain the treasure without immersing oneself in the cesspool at the bottom of which it lies. Most people, however, get frightened off by the stench and never begin the process. Many who begin the process do not follow through or are not allowed to. In the former case, they are bought off with a smaller treasure, mistaking it for the great one; in the latter case, society intervenes to halt the process.

Farber: I take it you've read Carl Jung?

Frank: Yes, and Freud, too.

Farber: Freud didn't have much faith in human potential.

Frank: Right, but you see, I wanted to understand his approach, and besides I didn't know that until I had read some of his writings. Between the two, I much preferred Jung's ideas. Freud, when he looked inside himself saw only a cesspool. Jung, looking within, saw not just the cesspool but in its murky depths, the treasure.

Freud, I believe, was correct when he said that dreams were "the royal road to the unconscious", but his interpretations were wrong: he didn't probe nearly deep enough. Had he, as Jung was more successful in doing, he would have found their spiritual essence. Freud got to the level of sexuality and power-grabbing. But at that point the inner phase of his journey ended and its outer phase began as he tried to persuade others that what he had discovered was the great treasure.

As I said, Jung went further than Freud in his understanding of the unconscious. Jung viewed the unconscious as a positive, creative force. Unlike Freud who saw dreams as merely the expression of unfulfilled drives for power and sex, Jung recognized that dreams also had a moral and spiritual dimension, that one of their major functions was to guide us onto and along the path of right living. Towards the end of his life, he dared to write what he probably had long believed that humanity "had forgotten the ancient fact that God speaks chiefly through dreams and visions", which is, of course, a major teaching of the leading western religions.

It's worth noting that the Hebrew words for dream and vision have the same root. In English, a vision is a dream than takes place while we're awake, while a dream is a vision that occurs when we're asleep. The former is very rare, while the latter is universally experienced. Ordinarily, it's difficult to relate to individuals who've had visions, especially these days, when in the psychiatric view visions are hallucinations, the hallmark symptom of schizophrenia. Of course, the Bible is filled with individuals who reportedly had visions, and it's easier to relate to these figures as people like you and me if you keep in mind that the words dream and vision are used almost interchangeable and that often what were spoken of as visions were more likely to have been dreams. The Bible, at least in the English translation, also used the word vision in another sense, to mean understanding and foresight as in the well-known verse, "Where there is no vision, the people perish." How little has changed since then! But people are yearning for change, a changed outlook, a

changed world, not so much for a new world
order as for a new world.

Joining the Movement

Farber: So how long was it before you got involved in the
               movement, which, I guess, at that point was called
               the "mental patients' liberation movement"?

Frank: That's getting a little ahead of the story. My release
               from Twin Pines Hospital was followed by a six-
               year period of intense study which ended in
               1969. Early that year, my friend Leo Hills moved
               his art gallery to a new location in downtown San
               Francisco, and he asked me to help him out in
               the gallery for a few weeks. I ended up working
               there for a year, first as a salesman, and then as
               the salesman/manager.
                  Because I did fairly well, I decided to open my
               own gallery and was fortunate to get a five-year
               lease at a fair rent on a store on the fringe of San
               Francisco's gallery district. But the gallery, which
               I opened in 1970, never worked out as a business
               project. It did, however, get me back into the
               workaday world where I could test myself. People
               would visit the gallery and we'd talk—and not
               only about art. Whenever I saw an opening, I'd
               discuss with them psychiatry/anti-psychiatry,
               sometimes distributing copies of articles critical
               of psychiatry.
                  All the while I continued my studies, mostly
               about psychiatry. Occasionally, I would express
               my views in letters to newspaper and magazine
               editors, few of which were published. One of
               these letters went to the editor of the *New York
               Times Book Review,* which in 1970 had reviewed
               a book by dissident psychiatrist Thomas Szasz.
               My letter criticized the review and supported
               Szasz's position. I sent a copy of this letter to
               Szasz. The *Times* didn't publish my letter, but
               Szasz sent me back a very nice note and that
               began a correspondence which soon turned into a
               friendship.

I had first heard about Szasz in 1964, a year after being released from Twin Pines. While in the San Francisco Public Library one day I had stumbled across a copy of *Harper's,* in which there was an article he had written. I could hardly believe what I read. Here was a psychiatrist—of all people—clearly explaining the truth about psychiatric oppression and 'mental illness'. I thought to myself, this man is writing precisely what I believed, although my critique was not nearly as well formulated. Immediately, I began reading as many of his books and articles as I could get hold of. Among the books of his I read at that time were *The Myth of Mental Illness* and *Law, Liberty, and Psychiatry.* By 1970, I had not only become thoroughly familiar with his views on psychiatry, freedom, and responsibility but had incorporated them into my own way of thinking.

Farber: In what ways did your thinking differ from Szasz's?

Frank: There were some differences but they were minor. On the important matters concerning psychiatry, we see eye to eye. Szasz believes that 'mental illness' is a myth that disguises and makes palatable "the bitter pill of moral conflicts in human relations". As he once phrased it, mental illness "has no meaning beyond its consequences." By "consequences" he meant that a psychiatrist's labelling someone mentally ill could result in that person's being committed and subjected to forced psychiatriatric 'treatment'. In other words, 'mental illness' is more a political than a medical term.

'Schizophrenia', 'depression', 'manic depression', and the like, are medicalized slur words used against those who won't or can't do what their families and society want them to. Szasz once said that being called a 'schizophrenic' by a psychiatrist today is like being called a Jew in Nazi Germany 50 years ago: it means 'garbage', take them away, get rid or them.

It's also like being called during the Middle Ages a 'heretic', which could result in the victim's being put on the rack or burned at the stake. Of course, we've come a long way since then; instead of burning bodies at the stake in the village square to intimidate the public by demonstrating what lay in store for those who don't stay in line, we burn brains with electroshock and occasionally televise a sanitized version of the procedure with the same end in view.

Farber: Were you influenced by Laing at that time?

Frank: No, he came on the scene for me a little later, toward the end of the 1960s when *The Politics of Experience* was published. Szasz played a much more important role in the development of my thinking about psychiatry than Laing, who, in my view, did not take a strong enough stand against involuntary psychiatry and never invalidated the 'medical model of mental illness' (the notion that 'mental illness is a disease like any other disease'), although he chipped away at it somewhat.

One of his important contributions was to popularize the idea that so-called 'schizophrenic behavior' was often a survival strategy developed by people in 'no-win' situations. He believed that people in such situations, when responded to with respect and kindness (or at least tolerance), instead of psychiatric labels, humiliation and incarceration, could go on to become better, freer, human beings. But Laing didn't always practice what he taught: I've heard that on occasion he would lock up people in psychiatric facilities, which, as you know, I'm wholly opposed to.

Farber: Were you seeing a therapist at this time?

Frank: No, no! While still locked up, I had told the psychiatrists that I would accept 'outpatient therapy' upon my release, and arrangements were made for me to see some psychoanalyst in San Francisco. But I was lying. I was under duress; they could have resumed shocking me; my life was hanging in the balance. Many people died from insulin-coma 'treatment'. A 1941 study I later ran across while I was researching my book, *The History of Shock Treatment,* reported a five percent death rate from the insulin-coma procedure then being administered in U.S. state hospitals. You do whatever is necessary in a situation like that. I didn't consider myself under any obligation to the psychiatrists to keep my word, no more than I would have had I given my word to the Gestapo while being tortured or threatened with torture. So I never called the psychoanalyst I had agreed to visit.

These white-jacketed brownshirts also wanted me to continue taking the psychiatric drugs they had started me on at Twin Pines. Even while I was there I hadn't been overly co-operative as far as these drugs were concerned. I remember the nurses occasionally checking my mouth when they suspected that I was 'cheeking' their drugs. Cheeking—I didn't know the term at the time—means storing a pill in your cheek while pretending to swallow it and later spitting it out. It was a legitimate suspicion for I would always avoid swallowing these drugs when I thought I could get away with it. The psychiatrist gave me a mess of pills when I was let out, and the first chance I had I flushed them down the toilet where I thought they belonged. This was before I had become aware of the harm pollutants do to the environment.

Once released, I never saw any therapists for 'therapy'. Actually, on one occasion I did see psychoanalyst Reider, my parents' agent. It was a few weeks after my release and my parents had let me know that I was to see him. The threat was implicit but clear: my refusal to see him could lead to my being recommitted.

So one day I kept an appointment with Reider at his office near Mount Zion Hospital in San Francisco. The furniture was Victorian; the place, dark. I remember very little of what was said, but the impression of a cold, distant, bitter man lingers with me. The meeting lasted about 20 minutes. There wasn't much communication. When I asked him about the memory problems I was having, he didn't respond. Again I asked, and

again he was silent. I may have asked him a third
time, with the same result. I remember my puz-
zlement at his not answering my question.

Only a few years later, after reading more
about psychoanalysis, did I discover that silence
was a ploy analysts sometimes used when they
don't want to answer a particular question: it was
their way of establishing dominance in the 'psychoanalytic relationship'. What I saw as rudeness
was for him probably an exercise in one-up-
manship. Soon after this exchange, he dismissed
me with a weak handshake. As I said goodbye, I
looked him in the eye; with a blank expression on
his face, he looked away. That was the last contact I had with him except once years later I met
him on the bus. Our eyes met for a moment. The
blank expression was still there. He died two
years ago.

That meeting in Reider's office was my last
'therapy' session. I suppose it could be said that
my attitude towards therapy was unduly colored
by my own experience with Reider and other
'therapists'. But I don't think so. I've since met a
number of therapists, who I've personally liked
and respected, some of whom I count among my
friends. I just don't believe in therapy as a medical enterprise. First of all, using the word therapy
implies that the person in therapy has a disease,
which in turn validates what I believe is a false
model. Furthermore, the benefit people derive
from therapy is mostly a matter of belief or faith.
In that sense, therapy is like religion: for those
who believe in it, it can do wonders. People also
may benefit from a therapist's showing concern
on hearing about their problems or it may happen that the therapist is able to come up with
some good advice in problem-solving or in helping the individual to understand him- or herself
better. But that's just counseling, and it has much
more to do with the counselor's wisdom and
compassion than with medicine or science.

I think a lot of people fool themselves about
the nature of their difficulties when they 'go into

therapy'. There's no disease here; they're not crazy, they're not going crazy. Such individuals have, in Szasz's term, "problems in living" or, from Laing's perspective, they're going through a spiritual crisis of some sort.

As I understand it, what they need above all is to confront themselves honestly, pinpoint the difficulties in their life situation, and work toward their resolution consciously and actively. They also need to transcend their small selves and live their lives on a higher moral plane. It's not a question of adjusting themselves to society: they need to transform themselves, and one of the best ways to begin the process is to spend a lot of time alone with themselves—at home, while jogging, or out in the woods,—meditating and thinking, especially about the possibility of change in their values, goals, lifestyle, relationships, job, and politics. Jesus said, Go into your closet and shut the door! Thoreau withdrew into his garret "determined to meet himself face to face sooner or later." And more recently, expressing the same theme, Arthur Schlesinger, Jr., wrote, "Everything that matters in our intellectual and moral life begins with an individual confronting his own mind and conscience in a room by himself."

To help us focus on the important issues, reading can be a useful tool. I mean serious reading, such as the Bible, Lao Tzu's *Way of Life,* Joseph Campbell's *Hero with a Thousand Faces,* and the writings of Emerson, Thoreau, Gandhi, and Martin Luther King, to name a few. In this last regard, even therapists have a contribution to make. People don't have to pay exorbitant fees and stay 'in therapy' for years to benefit from their teachings. Valuable lessons can be learned from reading inexpensive paperbacks by Szasz, Laing, Jung, and even Freud, but these authors, like others generally, must be approached with a critical eye: none of them has all the answers and readers must be as ready to reject as accept their views. What the best authors have to offer are not pat answers but provocative thoughts which stim-

ulate readers to do their own thinking and make
their own judgments.

If outside assistance is needed, family members, friends and acquaintances, self-help groups
are sometimes available. But the keynote here is
self-reliance, and if no one is available to assist
you, as may well be the case, then you have to be
prepared to go it alone. Even if outside support is
available, however, there are still certain legs of
the journey that must be undertaken unaided,
alone and away from people either periodically or
for an indeterminate period over a continuous
stretch of time.

There are dangers involved in this, not only
from within yourself but also from society. Regarding the internal risks, there may be periods of
confusion and loneliness, here the crucial factors
is self-trust and perseverance—you've just got to
tough it out. Regarding the external risks, Emerson said it best in one of his lectures, "Whoso
goes to walk alone, accuses the whole world; he
declares all to be unfit to be his companions; it is
very uncivil, nay, insulting; Society will retali-
ate." In our time, psychiatry is one of society's
most formidable instruments of retaliation.

Therapeutic 'Success'

Farber: Would you talk about the factors that account for the
success some therapists have in assisting people
who are in therapy?

Frank: I'm not so sure that they have that much success, and
how do you measure success anyway? Electro-
shock specialists, for example, claim a 'success'
rate of 80–90 percent for their procedure, but
they themselves set the criteria for improvement
and for the most part do the evaluating. Even by
their own success criteria, there is very little evidence demonstrating greater benefit beyond the
one-month period following 'treatment' than
would be obtained if the subjects had been left

alone or had been given sham-electroshock treatments. The short-run nature of electroshock 'success', if you want to call it that, was reaffirmed in a 1984 study undertaken by a well-known electroshock specialist who reported a 20–50 percent 'relapse' rate within six months after the completion of an electroshock series.

I know you're talking about psychotherapy, but the problems facing those who try to determine the effectiveness of various psychiatric treatments are similar. Actually, from my point of view, it's an impossible task, for there is no way to measure the effectiveness of a treatment for a non-existent disease.

Instead I'll discuss what there is about psychotherapy as conducted by psychiatrists or medically-oriented psychologists that makes it 'work', or at least seem to work, for those who say they benefit from it. The patient's readiness to believe therapy is going to be helpful is fundamental. The therapist's belief in therapy and in him- or herself is of almost equal importance.

When psychotherapy works, it's often, to use a psychiatric term, a case of *folie à deux,* that is, both parties share the same illusion: the therapist and the patient validate their own and the other's roles, the one as healer and the other as sick person. Any relationship, in which each party's illusion reinforces the other's, is going to be somewhat 'successful', at least until one of the parties becomes disillusioned. Another factor is the therapists' understanding and compassion or their ability to project those qualities. People with problems usually respond well to such traits regardless of background and training of the person whose traits they are.

But as I've said, the key seems to be the individual's faith in the process or in the therapist, who in effect is acting like a priest, a secular priest. Of course, what I'm talking about now is the voluntary therapeutic relationship. If it's a forced relationship, that's an altogether different story. When that's the case, the benefit is strictly one-sided: the therapists derive power, status, and money from the relationship, while the so-called patients lose their autonomy and dignity while being cowed into submission through intimidation and/or the physical, brain-disabling 'treatments'.

Fighting the System

Farber: When did you first get involved in *Madness Network News?*

Frank: That was in 1972. The first issue came out in 1972, and I contributed an article to the second issue.

Farber: But there was already a mental patient liberation organization, right?

Frank: Yes, the first group was organized in Portland, Oregon, and was called the "Insane Liberation Front".

Farber: But there was no group in San Francisco before *Madness Network News.*

Frank: Actually, *MNN* was preceded by a small group of psychiatric survivors and mental-health professionals, including my friend psychiatrist David Richman, who later wrote *Dr. Caligari's Psychiatric Drugs,* an excellent informational booklet based in part on regular columns he had contributed to *MNN.* In 1971 or 1972, this group had organized an educational seminar, a weekend program in the Bay Area, where they discussed madness, mostly in Laingian terms, and the need for alternatives to traditional psychiatric treatment.

Farber: Well, Laing had a tremendous impact on campuses in the late sixties.

Frank: That's true. Unfortunately, that impact didn't extend to the mental hospitals, where it would have really counted. In those places, everything went along more or less as it had always gone along. The problem was that some people paid lip service to Laing, just as others—with some overlap—paid lip service to Szasz, but in terms of the way psychiatry was being practiced, very little changed. Since the early 1970s, the situation has actually worsened: psychiatrists more than ever before rely on mystification, threats, drugs, electroshock, and what is at the heart of this approach, the biological view of mental illness as a physical disease, and more specifically, a brain disease.

And nowadays, fewer and fewer psychiatrists even refer, let alone pay lip service, to Szasz and Laing. For example, the index of the latest edition of a standard psychiatric textbook doesn't even list Szasz; the same textbook in an earlier edition, published in the 1970s, carried more than 30 index citations for him.

Szasz has been dropped into psychiatry's "memory hole", which George Orwell in his classic *Nineteen Eighty-Four* described as the repository for those persons and facts the knowledge of which Party historian-revisionists thought would be harmful to the Party's current interests. They were, in effect, using shock treatment on their history books, a kind of bookwashing, the application of brainwashing to history. Brainwashing, too, is what shock treatment is really all about. As one psychiatrist described his post-intensive electroshock "patients," "their minds seem like clean slates upon which we can write."

Many interesting parallels, incidentally, can be drawn between inquisitorial psychiatry and Orwell's dystopia: for example, diagnostic terminology (or psychspeak) is 'newspeak', psychiatrists are 'thought police', and delusions are 'thoughtcrimes'. Winston, Orwell's prototypical outsider, was even electroshocked in the course of bringing him back into the fold, which was merely a question of his 'learning to think as they thought', or more accurately, his learning not to think at all.

Yes, Big Brother is alive and well. For all we know, Orwell shaped him in the image of the modern psychiatrist. Like Big Brother, psychiatrists also appear regularly on television. They don't dominate the screen as he did, just the conversation, with Phil, Oprah, Sally, and other talk-show hosts who treat them, because of their authority, with automatic reverence.

Farber: How long were you involved with *MNN?*

Frank: On and off for about 12 years. It was last published in 1985. One of the highlights of that association was the publication in 1974 of the *Madness Network News Reader* by Glide Publications of San Francisco. It is an anthology of writings mostly from *MNN* and offers a good overview of some of the movement's early thinking.

Also in 1974, the Network Against Psychiatric Assault, or NAPA, was formed. Wade Hudson and I, its co-founders, decided to start the group because *MNN,* where we had worked together and had become friends, was not by itself sufficient for the political work we believed was necessary to further our cause which was, and continues to be, the abolition of involuntary psychiatry.

We wanted to confront organized psychiatry politically, and almost immediately began organizing a campaign to halt the use of electroshock by force or without informed consent at the Langley Porter Psychiatric Hospital at the University of California in San Francisco. The demonstrations and rallies NAPA organized at Langley Porter were covered extensively by the media and were embarrassing to the hospital's staff and the university, which didn't relish its being pictured as a place where people were being dragged off for electroshock.

There were also demonstrations at San Francisco's St. Mary's Hospital, a general hospital which had a psych ward. We had been angered by reports that the ward, in addition to the standard forced drugging, was also using what was called 'harassment therapy', which involved forcing psychiatric inmates to do degrading chores like scrubbing the floor with a toothbrush. The psychiatrists there were also using a particularly vicious form of physical restraint called 'sheeting', in which inmates were immobilized for hours on end in tightly wrapped bedsheets.

Farber: It's amazing how they could get away with such obvious cruelty!

Frank: Well, psychiatrists are still getting away with similarly dehumanizing techniques; four-point restraints are available in most psychiatric wards, coerced drugging is still commonplace, and lately there's been a resurgence in the use of electroshock.

Along with the demonstrations, we lobbied vigorously for legislation that would restrict the use of electroshock and psychosurgery in California. Toward this end we were successful in enlisting the support of Assembly Member John Vasconcellos. The bill he introduced early in 1974 was passed later that year but was immediately challenged in the courts by the psychiatric profession. Later, a California Supreme Court ruling forced Vasconcellos to revise the bill and it finally went into effect in 1977. The 'Vasconcellos Bill', as it came to be known, proved to be a landmark in the field of psychiatric law. It not only effectively eliminated the use of psychosurgery in California, but also served as a model for legislation restricting electroshock elsewhere: since its passage, more than 30 states have enacted similar legislation.

Farber: What other activities was Network Against Psychiatric Assault engaged in?

Frank: NAPA published two booklets, one was entitled *Forced Treatment Equals Torture,* the other was an earlier, much briefer, mimeographed version of my book *The History of Shock Treatment.* We also sponsored educational forums and seminars. My art gallery, being centrally located, was very useful during NAPA's early stages for it became the site of some of these forums and also our organizational meetings. In 1974, we packed into the gallery as many as 90 or 100 people for forums on psychiatric drugs, electroshock, legal issues, the oppression of women and children by psychiatry, and the like.

In the spring of that year, we held a public meeting attended by about 250 people at the Glide Church to inform the public about the issues and rally support for our political activities. In January 1975, Glide also became the site of an address by Szasz before about 1,200 people. He spoke on "The Myth of Psychotherapy", which a few years later he used as the title for what I believe is one of his finest books.

The storm we had raised about Langley Porter's use of electroshock resulted in public hearings in San Francisco. Supervisor Quentin Keep of the Board of Supervisors conducted the hearing in January 1976. That hearing, in combination with the then newly passed electroshock legislation led to a two-year moratorium on ECT use in San Francisco.

In July of the same year we carried out a 30-day sleep-in demonstration at Governor Jerry Brown's office at the State Capitol in Sacramento to protest conditions in state hospitals, particularly the forced drugging of inmates and their being made to work without pay—under the guise of 'occupational therapy'. In 1976 we also held protest demonstrations at San Francisco's Federal Building against the return of psychosurgery which the federal government was in the process of sanctioning. It was a very busy and productive period for NAPA.

In the early 1980s, NAPA, which by then had moved its offices to Berkeley, across the bay from San Francisco, led demonstrations at Herrick Hospital, a notorious shock mill in Berkeley. These demonstrations sparked an all-day public hearing on electroshock before Berkeley's Human Relations and Welfare Commission (chaired by David Cunningham) in the spring of 1982. The testimony was overwhelmingly anti-shock—only two people, both psychiatrists, spoke out for shock, the others, more than 40 people were strongly opposed to its use.

The hearing was the springboard, later that year, for a successful referendum campaign to ban electroshock in Berkeley. The campaign was spearheaded by Ted Chabasinski, who had been electroshocked at New York's Bellevue Hospital in 1944 when he was six years old. More than 60 percent of Berkeley's citizens voted to criminalize the use of electroshock in their community. Unfortunately, a Superior Court summary judgment overturned the ban only a few weeks after it had gone into effect. The ruling was upheld on appeal right up to California's Supreme Court.

It's pretty clear that we've had our successes and our defeats. But that's not the way I measure the value of these and other activities. I see them as part of a larger picture of resistance to psychiatric tyranny that is taking place across the country and in other countries too—Canada, Britain, Holland, Germany, Italy, Australia, and New Zealand, among others.

The continental movement is reflected in the growth, beginning in the seventies, of a network of political groups made up of psychiatric survivors. For 12 years beginning in 1973 many of us from these groups met at the Annual Conference on Human Rights and Psychiatric Oppression in cities throughout the United States and once in Canada.

At these conferences we educated ourselves about psychiatric labelling and violence and how psychiatry depoliticizes and despiritualizes people, organized local demonstrations against particularly abusive practices, and in the last few conferences took part in acts of civil disobedience (CD) against offending psychiatric facilities and the American Psychiatric Association itself.

The most memorable of these CDs took place at our 1982 conference in Toronto. Fifteen of us conducted a sit-in in the lobby at the Sheraton Centre Hotel where the APA was holding its Annual Meeting. After we had spent about two hours protesting against electroshock and forced drugging, the police arrived and soon escorted

us—some of us were carried off—to waiting pad-
dy wagons. We were finally released from jail
several hours later, but only after coming up with
bail money—about $50 for each of us.

I don't know how to estimate the impact this
event had on organized psychiatry and on the
community, but there's no doubt about the tremendous unifying effect it had on the participants and our supporters. As one of those
arrested, I can attest to this personally. I look
forward to the time when we in the movement
will once again engage in acts of civil disobedience as a rallying point for movement activists,
to draw the public's attention to abusive psychiatric practices, and also to awaken the consciences
of the perpetrators themselves.

Another benefit we derived from our annual
conferences was that we formed many solid
friendships among ourselves and made alliances
with other human-rights organizations. In recent
years, the emphasis in our movement has
switched from confrontational politics of the sort
I have been describing to self-help organizing. I
believe the movement's next phase will see a
joining together of these two approaches and a
snowballing of participation by psychiatric survivors, and eventually the public at large.

The Crime of Electroshock

Farber: Lately, I've been reading about the electroshock hearings in San Francisco. What brought on the hear-
ings and how do they fit into the overall picture?

Frank: Back in April of 1990, Vince Bielski wrote a cover
story for the *San Francisco Bay Guardian* about
electroshock's "quiet comeback", raising questions about the procedure's benefits and dangers
and possible human-rights violations in connection with its use in Bay Area hospitals. He also
reported that plans were afoot at three San Francisco hospitals to resume using ECT.

The article alerted Supervisor Angela Alioto of San Francisco's board of supervisors who called for public hearings before the City Services Committee, which she chairs, to investigate the issue. Consequently, three hearings, lasting a total of about 12 hours, were held between November of 1990 and February of 1991.

Other than several electroshock specialists and other psychiatrists and physicians, the witnesses roundly condemned the procedure. Most of the pro-ECT witnesses were from a special ad hoc committee of the Northern California Psychiatric Society (an APA branch) which also assigned a public-relations person to help present its case. Included in the NCPS packet distributed at the first hearing was the ad hoc committee's catechism on ECT, which claimed that "there is no brain-tissue destruction" from ECT.

But the anti-ECT forces, which included psychiatrist Peter Breggin, author of *Electroshock: Its Brain-Disabling Effects,* who had flown out from Bethesda, Maryland for the hearing; neurologist John Friedberg, author of *Shock Treatment Is Not Good For Your Brain;* former psychoanalyst Jeffrey Moussaieff Masson, author of *Against Therapy;* psychologist Bob Morgan, editor of *Electroshock: The Case Against;* psychiatrist David Richman, author of *Dr. Caligari's Psychiatric Drugs;* lawyers and advocates; and electroshock survivors, their relatives and friends, were not only far more numerous, but were far more persuasive than the electroshock proponents.

Among other things, critics testified about human-rights abuses—that is, electroshock administered by force, coercion or without informed consent—how women and the elderly were being electroshocked in disproportionately large numbers, about ECT-caused memory loss and brain injury, and how the procedure robs people of their humanity and diminishes their ability to function in society.

Soon after the hearings, in March, the board of supervisors passed a non-binding resolution, later

signed by Mayor Art Agnos, which stated the
Board's opposition to the use and financing of
ECT, and urged the state legislature to tighten up
the informed-consent process in the present ECT
law. The resolution didn't go nearly as far as we'd
have liked, but it was the first time a major U.S.
city had taken such a stand. The resolution, together with the hearings, also generated a good
deal of media coverage, including reports on CBS
evening news and CNN, and thus informed many
people about the dangers of ECT and the fact
that at least in some quarters its use is being
actively opposed. The board of supervisors's action also demonstrated the legitimacy of govern-
mental intervention in psychiatric practices
where public safety and human rights are at issue.

It's hard to tell what the ripple effect of these
activities will be, but as other ECT hearings have
demonstrated, one thing leads to another. Only
weeks after passage of the resolution, Assembly
Member Gil Ferguson introduced a bill that
would further restrict the use of ECT in California.

Still there's no cause for complacency. The
three San Francisco hospitals that a year ago were
planning to resume ECT, as reported in the *Bay
Guardian,* are now actually using the procedure.
San Francisco now has four electroshock hospitals. Ironically, and tragically, the city named for
St. Francis, that gentlest of human beings, has
become a major center for electroshock, one of
the most vicious techniques ever devised for bru-
talizing and dehumanizing human beings. I believe the trend in San Francisco toward
increasing electroshock-use represents fairly what
is happening across the country and that this
trend is a direct consequence of the American
Psychiatric Association's giant promotional campaign on behalf of ECT.

In 1990 the APR came out with a task-force
report, *The Practice of Electroconvulsive Therapy,*
hailing ECT technique modifications which they
claimed make the procedure safe and effective

and recommending electroshock use not only for "depression" but also for "schizophrenia" and "manic-depression", and for children and the elderly who are supposedly "mentally ill". The report also minimizes ECT-caused memory loss and advises psychiatrists and hospitals that "in light of the available evidence, 'brain damage' need not be included as a potential risk" on the informed consent form. With much fanfare, these outright lies are being passed off as scientific truths. To announce publication of the task-force study, the APA even held a press conference, on which the Associated Press ran an uncritical story.

Farber: But how do you respond to psychiatrists who claim that ECT is very different today compared with what it used to be. I've heard them say, for example, the public has a false picture of ECT based on that scene in 'One Flew Over the Cuckoo's Nest', in which Jack Nicholson is seen in obvious pain, gritting his teeth and thrashing about during an electroconvulsion?

Frank: It is true that there have been changes in the method of administering electroshock, but they have been mostly cosmetic. The most important of these changes were introduced during the mid-1950s. Around that time many ECT specialists started using anesthetics and muscle-relaxants to reduce fear, pain, and the risk of bone complications. The depiction of ECT in 'Cuckoo's Nest', by the way, was based on Ken Kesey's observations in the early 1960s at a California VA hospital where muscle-relaxants were not being used.

Without the muscle-relaxants, the procedure caused bone and spinal fractures in 15–25 percent of ECT subjects. The muscle-relaxants have virtually eliminated that problem. They also made the procedure easier to administer and much less distressing to watch; other than some twitching in the hands and feet, little body movement is observed.

With electroshock, however the most significant activity, takes place out of sight, in the subject's brain which experiences an electrical storm at least as severe as it would without the relaxants. I say "at least as severe" because the use of these drugs involves a trade-off: the anesthetics and muscle-relaxants not only carry their own risks, including death, but they also raise the individual's convulsive threshold so that more electric current is needed to induce the convulsion, and it is the current which is the procedure's most brain-damaging component. That's something the ECT supporters don't talk about publicly, but they sometimes mention it, without emphasis, in their literature.

Another modification deals with electrode placement. Formerly, placement of the two electrodes, through which the current is passed, was always on the temples, with the frontal-lobe area of the brain receiving the brunt of the assault— just as it does in a lobotomy operation. In the late 1960s unilateral ECT was introduced as an alternative to the old method which was called bilateral ECT. In unilateral ECT one electrode is placed on a temple, the other above the back of the neck on the same side of the head. Almost from the start this new technique was the source of controversy among the push-button psychiatrists.

The unilateralists claimed unilateral ECT caused less memory loss; the bilateralists claimed that, while that may be true, it was less effective than bilateral ECT and therefore required more 'treatments'. One of the bilateralists went so far as to say that unilateral ECT's "failure to cure was in direct proportion to its avoidance of memory loss". In so stating, he was unwittingly supporting one of the major charges ECT critics have been making against all electroshock: namely, that it 'works' by causing memory loss: ECT subjects forget what had been troubling them or what they had been saying or doing that had troubled others and are thus perceived as 'improved'. Of course, this is no real solution to any problem; it's like sweeping dirt under the rug. In return for this so-called improvement, ECT subjects must suffer brain damage for as every neurologist knows one of the surest signs of brain damage is memory loss.

To electroshock someone is not merely a matter of malpractice: it's a crime. Because the brain damage it causes hampers one's ability to think, electroshock violates the freedom of thought principle implicit in the 'freedom of speech' clause of the Bill of Rights' First Amendment. It's also a crime against the spirit. Look at it this way, If the body is the temple of the spirit, as I believe, then the brain may be seen as the inner sanctum of the body, the holiest of holy places. To invade, violate and injure the brain, as electroshock unfailingly does, is a desecration of the soul.

And the public is buying into this outrageous practice. Duped again, just as it was in the 1940s and 1950s when psychiatrists were ballyhooing lobotomies as a means of restoring 'the insane' to 'normalcy' and 'productive living'. As most people now know, the lobotomies produced only vegetables. But the situation with regards to electroshock is much worse today because many more people are effected. All told, *only* 50,000 people in the U.S. were lobotomized, whereas an estimated 100,000 people are now being electroshocked in this country *every year*.

As you can see, we've got our work cut out for us. But we have made some progress, mostly in getting the word out and in laying the groundwork for future political activity.

How to Change the System

Farber: All that's pretty nebulous. Specifically, what can people do right now?

Frank: Lots of things. To name a few: writing letters to the media, and to local, state, and Congressional representatives in order to protest about particular

psychiatric abuses—perhaps calling for public
hearings; lobbying for laws that prevent psychiatrists from violating the rights of others; and getting signatures on petitions to gain citizen
support.

Also informing yourself about the issues—
that's so fundamental it might better go at the
head of the list. It's virtually impossible to persuade people to change their minds about something that's important to them when you yourself
are uninformed. To have any chance at all, you
need to be knowledgeable, and to become knowledgeable, you have to start listening to and talking with others who are.

It also helps to read up on the subject. Psychiatric survivors Judi Chamberlin, Janet Gotkin,
and Kate Millet have written superb books about
their experiences and the political issues surrounding psychiatric practice—*On Our Own, Too
Much Anger, Too Many Tears,* and *The Loony Bin
Trip,* respectively. The writings of Szasz, Breggin,
and Masson are extremely useful. *Dr. Caligari's
Psychiatric Drugs, Madness Network News Reader,* and *The History of Shock Treatment* can also
be helpful in understanding the nature of psychiatry. *Dendron News,* a quality journal which
David Oaks publishes in Eugene, Oregon, provides on ongoing account of movement opinion
and activities.

As I've already mentioned, there's a role in our
movement for civil disobedience and nonviolence, as practiced by Gandhi and King. But it
takes organization to move in that direction. So
people need to begin organizing themselves in a
more focussed way, with specific political objec-
tives. Incidentally, CD is an excellent way to help
build an organization. Actually the two feed off
each other: with organization you can conduct
CD; with CD you can recruit people to the movement. The same could be said for protest demonstrations generally.

It's important that as many psychiatric survivors as possible be involved. There are literally

millions of us survivors of psychiatric dehumanization. That there are so few of us who are fighting back is a sad fact. It is also testimony to the effectiveness of psychiatry as an instrument of social control. The vast majority of us—in shame, out of not knowing, from fear (of being ostracized, reinstitutionalized, or getting fired), or because of treatment-caused disability—have chosen or have been forced to remain on the sidelines. Now is the time to step forward and participate in the struggle to win human rights in psychiatry.

I know there are many survivors who feel hopeless about the possibilities of bringing about meaningful change given the current political atmosphere, but that is a poor excuse for inaction. That we can do only a little is no excuse for doing nothing at all. And even if we can do only a little, that little can make a difference, and sometimes a big difference, just as each grain of sand contributes to the scale's being tipped in one direction or another. I would encourage everyone to do what they can with what they've got.

I would encourage psychiatric survivors and others to consider the entire social picture of which psychiatry forms only a part. Psychiatry is locked into society as a whole; it is in fact a microcosm of that society, one of many interlocking institutions which together form a self-perpetuating system.

One aspect of the system is that people are treated as objects to be used and manipulated in the service of a social system which is dominated by a relatively small minority. Instead of the system serving people, people are forced to serve the system. Any meaningful change in the system must be comprehensive and it must restructure the system's moral underpinnings. The change must be in the way we relate to each other, and it must include more caring and respect for one another and a more equal sharing of political power and economic resources.

We have the means right now to provide a living wage for everyone who wants to work, but our priorities are all wrong; we have put profits ahead of people. As a result of which, millions are unjustly, needlessly, and senselessly deprived of what is a basic, albeit mostly unrecognized, human right. Reforming psychiatry in isolation, without bringing about these other changes, will not work; some other repressive force would merely step in and take its place, just as organized psychiatry 300 years ago replaced the Inquisition.

We psychiatric survivors, first as human beings, need to work on ourselves and with others to transform our society. We need to embrace the poor, women, and racial and ethnic minorities, indeed all the disadvantaged and disillusioned from every walk of life among all the peoples of the Earth. We need to sound a rallying cry which will bring together all humanity.

✧ ✧ ✧ ✧ ✧ ✧ ✧ ✧ ✧ ✧ ✧

Appendix 1
Required Reading for Revolters

Thomas Szasz, *The Manufacture of Madness: A Comparative Study of the Inquisition and the Mental Health Movement* (New York: Harper and Row, 1970). This may be the single most important book on the subject. It is a beautiful, profound elegy, an impassioned defense of freedom, a searing attack on the psychiatric inquisitors and their religion of medical science, a meditation on the spiritual crisis of humanity and a challenge to all of us to transcend the "existential cannibalism" that has characterized the human species for centuries. Szasz notes astutely that psychiatric 'diagnosis' "constitutes the initial act of social validation and invalidation, pronounced by the high priest of modern scientific religion, the psychiatrist; it justifies the expulsion of the sacrificial scapegoat, the mental patient, from the community." This book helped to establish Szasz as one of the great moral figures of our century.

Thomas Szasz, *The Myth of Mental Illness: Foundations of a Theory of Personal Conduct* (New York: Hoeber-Harper, 1961). Szasz's first book on the topic.

Thomas Szasz, *Insanity: The Idea and Its Consequences* (New York: Wiley, 1987). A systematic answer to Szasz's critics over the years.

Thomas Szasz, *A Lexicon of Lunacy: Metaphoric Malady, Moral Responsibility, and Psychiatry* (New Brunswick, NJ: Transaction, 1993).

R.D. Laing, *The Politics of Experience* (New York: Pantheon, 1967). This is Laing's best and boldest statement. Unfortunately, he spent the rest of his career defending, qualifying, and even apologizing for this work. Next to *The Manufacture of Madness,* it is the most important book on the topic. Laing prophecies that if the human race survives the present "Age of Darkness", human beings of the future will look back on us with compassion and amusement: "They will see that what we call 'schizophrenia' was one of the forms in which, often through quite ordinary people, the light began to break through the cracks in our all-too-closed minds." Laing resumed elegantly, but

241

unsurely, the dialogue between reason and unreason, between the 'sane' and the mad, a dialogue that was stopped two centuries ago when madness was redefined as 'mental illness'. (I am wholeheartedly committed to carrying on this dialogue, and consequently to affirming the ontological validity of 'madness'.)

R.D. Laing and A. Esterson, *Sanity, Madness and Family* (New York: Basic Books, 1965). The main virtue of this book is its demonstration that the discourse of mad people makes sense.

R.D. Laing, *The Voice of Experience* (New York: Pantheon Books, 1982). Part I of the book contains some of Laing's best essays, Part II is of little interest to persons who are not obsessed with intrauterine experiences. Of particular interest is Laing's interpretation of a dialogue between a 'schizophrenic' and a famous psychoanalyst. Laing demonstrates that the former is far more eloquent, far more compassionate and more in touch with 'reality'.

R.D. Laing, *Wisdom, Madness and Folly: The Making of a Psychiatrist* (New York: McGraw Hill, 1985). Laing's last book, an exquisitely poetic swan-song by a man who died "disheartened" because he was so misunderstood by fellow intellectuals.

Erving Goffman, *Asylums: Essays on the Social Situation of Mental Patients and Other Inmates* (New York: Anchor Books, 1961). This book should have put the 'mental health' system out of business.

Peter Breggin, *Toxic Psychiatry: Why Therapy, Empathy, and Love Must Replace the Drugs, Electroshock, and Biochemical Theories of the 'New Psychiatry'* (New York: St. Martin's Press, 1991). This detailed book is an indispensable alternative textbook that counters the propaganda of modern psychiatry. Breggin himself is one of the few psychiatrists who has had the courage and the compassion to publicly denounce the psychiatric establishment and to ally himself with psychiatric survivors. In this book he documents the rise of the "psychopharmaceutical complex", a coalition of industries more resistant to change than the 'military industrial complex', and he discusses in detail the toxic effects of the most widely used psychiatric drugs.

Thomas Scheff, *Being Mentally Ill* (Chicago: Aldine, 1966).

Theodore Sarbin and James Mancuso, *Schizophrenia: Medical Diagnosis or Moral Verdict?* (New York: Pergamon, 1980).

D. Rosenhan, 'On Being Sane in Insane Places'. In Paul Watzlawick (ed.), *The Invented Reality* (New York: Norton, 1984).

Michel Foucault, *Madness and Civilization* (New York: Vintage, 1965).

Kate Millet, *The Loony-Bin Trip* (New York: Simon and Schuster, 1991). An absorbing and enlightening personal story. The epilogue is a brilliant and succinct defense of 'madness' as an expression of the imagination.

David Cohen (ed.), *Challenging the Therapeutic State: Critical Perspectives on Psychiatry and the Mental Health System* (*The Journal of Mind and Behavior*, P.O. Box 522, Village Station, New York, NY 10014. $18). A thorough 'postmodern' debunking of the medical model. Particularly recommended are articles by Leifer, Sarbin, Farber, Scull, Gergen, and Frank.

John Modrow, *How to Become a Schizophrenic: The Case Against Biological Psychiatry* (Apollyon Press, P.O. Box 5114, Everett, WA). Written by a bona fide 'schizophrenic'.

Jay Haley, *Leaving Home: The Therapy of Disturbed Young People* (New York: McGraw Hill, 1980). Haley argues that most 'therapists' have abandoned the pretense of helping to effect personal growth and have become social control agents.

Jeffrey Masson, *Against Therapy: Emotional Tyranny and the Myth of Psychological Healing* (New York: Atheneum, 1988). Debunks Freud and his disciples.

Judi Chamberlin, *On Her Own* (New York: Harper and Row, 1980). An astute critique of psychiatry by an ex-'mental patient' who became a human rights activist.

In order to understand how dehumanizing modern psychology is, it is necessary to compare it to a more exalted conceptions of what it means to be a human being:

Selected Writings of Ralph Waldo Emerson. Two essays in particular, *The Divinity School Address* and *The Over-Soul.* Emerson articulates Christ's sublime and grand vision of human potential, and he explicates the tragic misinterpretation of Christ's teachings promulgated by "historic Christianity".

Rabbi Abraham J. Heschel, *The Prophets: An Introduction* (New York: Harper and Row, 1962). A genuine religious perspective is concerned primarily not with mystical experience but with 'historical justice'. "Mystical experience is the illumination of an individual; historical justice is the illumination of all human beings, enabling the inhabitants of the world to learn righteousness."

Vladimir Solovyov, *The Meaning of Love* (West Stockbridge, MA: Lindisfarne Press, 1984) Solovyov lived from 1853 to 1900. I find him the most profound and prescient Christian theologian and visionary. He believed that romantic love was potentially the instrument for effecting the kind of spiritual transformation that would enable us to attain physical immortality and to realize the Kingdom of God on earth.

Robert McDermott (ed.), *The Essential Aurobindo* (New York: Schocken, 1973). Aurobindo Ghose ('Sri Aurobindo') was a Hindu philosopher and yogi (1878–1950), who wrote in English. He was one of the greatest sages who ever lived.

Other Resources:

Dendron. The best anti-psychiatric magazine in the country. For a free copy, write to: *Dendron,* P.O. Box 11284, Eugene, OR 97440.

National Association of Psychiatric Survivors, P.O. Box 618, Sioux Falls, SD 57101. Membership fee is $25.

To obtain legal aid against psychiatric abuse, write to the National Association of Protection and Advocacy, 220 Eye Street, N.E., Suite 150, Washington, DC 20001. Or call 202-546-8202.

Network Against Coercive Psychiatry. See Appendix 3.

For a one-hour video discussion featuring Kate Millett, Ron Leifer, Seth Farber, and Sally Clay, send $19.95 to: Proud Eye Productions, 44 Great Hill Road, New Town, CT 06470. (Allow 6–8 weeks for delivery.)

✧ ✧ ✧ ✧ ✧ ✧ ✧ ✧ ✧ ✧ ✧

Appendix 2
Why Deinstitutionalization Failed

> We will convince them that they can never be free because they are weak, vicious, worthless and rebellious. . . . In the end they will lay their freedom at our feet and say we don't mind being your slaves as long as you feed us.
> From "The Grand Inquisitor" in Dostoyevsky's *The Brothers Karamazov*

A large part of the business of institutional psychiatry consists of the manufacture and marketing of a culturally enveloping, socially validated, economically lucrative, delusional system. Institutional psychiatry has about as much interest in eliminating the phenomena it classifies as 'mental illness', as the military-industrial complex has in eliminating war and the threat of war. Its own existence requires the perpetuation of unhappiness and suffering and the continued adherence to ideologies that lead it to hinder rather than help individuals in their attempt to resolve problems in living.

Critics of institutional psychiatry have been marginalized and ignored for the last 30 years. A theoretical foundation exists for a paradigm shift; the literature countering the medical model is now voluminous. It includes not only critiques of the foundations of the disease model of human behavior, but accounts of therapeutic and social interventions that produce dramatic and remarkably successful outcomes in individuals who would have been classified as 'chronically mentally ill' by mainstream psychiatry. These alternative therapists include pioneers in the family therapy movement such as Salvador Minuchin, Jay Haley, Carl Whitaker, the Mental Research Institute, as well as a variety of approaches inspired by the work of the unconventional psychiatrist Milton H. Erickson. It should be noted that the family therapy movement was, for the most part, co-opted by institutional psychiatry before it had a chance to develop an independent identity.

In 1980, Theodore Sarbin and James Mancuso published *Schizophrenia: Medical Diagnosis or Moral Verdict,* in which they meticulously examined 20 years of research designed to prove that 'schizophrenia' is a disease that destroys the afflicted individual's intellectual and percep-

Reprinted with permission from Z magazine, April 1992.

tual capacities. They demonstrate that the research (published in psychiatry's most prestigious journals) is deficient, that the researchers had failed to come up with one single dependent variable to reliably distinguish 'schizophrenics' from 'normal' people. This book, already out of print, is not even mentioned in the neoconservative defense of institutional psychiatry, *Madness in the Streets,* by Raul Jean Isaac and Virginia Armat (Free Press, 1990. The senior author is a frequent contributor to *Commentary.*)

In the introduction to the Sarbin and Mancuso book, psychologist Leonard Krasner pinpoints the obstacles to humanitarian reforms within the mental health system: "It would be an interesting exercise in economics and occupational sociology to show in detail how schizophrenia as a disease metaphor has spawned thousands of jobs, not only for the psychiatric teams (psychiatrists, clinical psychologists and social workers, and other mental health employees), but also for the pharmaceutical, publishing, hospital supply and related industries. The first task of any industry is to perpetuate itself and then to expand."

Deinstitutionalization

The task force report of the American Psychiatric Association *The Practice of Electroconvulsive Therapy: Recommendations for Treating, Training, and Privileging* (1990) reveals the dishonesty and moral depravity to which psychiatry has sunk. I write "sunk" because the deinstitutionalization movement, despite its roots in economic exigencies, held high the promise of reintegrating individuals into the community who had previously been locked away for years in state mental hospitals. This movement, which began in 1955 and accelerated between 1965 and 1985, reduced the state inmate hospital population by more than three quarters.

The hope for a genuine transformation in policy was fuelled by intellectual ferment within psychiatry, symbolized by the publication of psychiatrist Thomas Szasz's book, *The Myth of Mental Illness* (1961). The idealism of some of the adherents of deinstitutionalization did not at the time seem to be totally naive. B. Alper wrote in a book edited by Y. Bakal, *Closing Correctional Institutions:* "By bringing [the mad and other deviants] back into the community, by enlisting the good will and the desire to serve, the ability to understand which is found in every neighborhood, we shall meet the challenge that such groups of persons present, and at the same time ease the financial burden of their confinement in fixed institutions."

These hopes were finally buried with the publication of *The Practice of Electroconvulsive Therapy.* Read in conjunction with *Madness in the Streets* which has won the accolades of the psychiatric community, we are given some sense of psychiatry's plans for those individuals it terms 'chronically mentally ill'. Psychiatry's response to the problem of 'mental illness' is no more enlightened and no less barbaric than the Nazis' response to the 'Jewish problem'.

These books are a response in large part to the failure of deinstitutionalization. In hindsight this failure appears to have been predictable. The movement began, as noted, as a result of economic factors. Historian Andrew Scull has documented that the process did not occur, as psychiatrists frequently claim, because newly discovered neuroleptic drugs cured 'mental illnesses', but was in response to "a broad expanse of social [federal] welfare programs, growing fiscal pressures on the states and the opportunity to transfer costs away from the state budget." Deinstitutionalized individuals were not integrated into the community but subsisted (and subsist) in private facilities, boarding rooms, single-room occupancy hotels, or, more frequently today, in the streets, because many of the private facilities have been torn down and converted into condominiums. Scull noted in his recent book *Decarceration* (1984): "It is only an illusion that patients who are placed in boarding or family care homes are in the community . . . These facilities are for the most part like small long-term state hospital wards, isolated from the community . . . Little effort is directed toward social and vocational rehabilitation . . . One is overcome by the depressing atmosphere not because of the physical appearance of the boarding home, but because of the passivity, isolation, and inactivity of the residents."

Why did deinstitutionalization fail to realize the ideal of integrating mental patients into society? Why was so little effort directed toward social and vocational rehabilitation as Scull noted? *Madness in the Streets* claims that it was an ill-conceived project from the start and that it had to fail because 'mental illness' is incapacitating and intractable and that this fact is not recognized by radical critics of psychiatry or by liberals in the mental health system who have been duped by these clever evil-doers.

If the arguments of *Madness in the Streets* were correct, ironically the book never would have been written. The book claims that the 'mentally ill' are genetically flawed, incorrigible, pathetic, incompetent and frequently antisocial and dangerous. Yet it also clearly regards the psychiatric survivors ("ex-mental patients") in the anti-psychiatry movement as "talented", "vigorous", shrewd, in short formidable opponents to psychiatry. But these individuals were seriously mentally ill by the criteria of psychiatry.

How did these pathetic, genetically flawed creatures develop into such a threat to psychiatry? (Virtually none of these individuals take the 'medication' they are reputed to need in order to function.) Of course neither the authors of *Madness* nor the numerous legions of psychiatrists who have lauded it as a definitive answer to the critics of psychiatry, are prepared to consider this question.

The answer is simple. These individuals were not afflicted by 'mental illness'. They went mad as a result of being overwhelmed by a number of problems: interpersonal, spiritual, economic. Madness is not necessarily a dysfunctional way of temporarily coping with stress. It is dysfunctional in a society in which vulnerable individuals are prey for the psychiatric-industrial complex. These independently-minded individuals escaped from the clutches of the 'mental health' system, found emotional support elsewhere, refused to accept that they were 'mentally ill', went back to school or work, engaged in the kind of meaningful activities that created a firm foundation for a sense of personal identity and self-worth, and became contributing members of the social order.

Deinstitutionalization failed because there were too many vested interests in its failure. Had it succeeded in reintegrating former 'mental patients' into society, it would have demonstrated the mythical nature of the idea of mental illness and would consequently have threatened the existence of both the psychiatric-industrial complex and the hegemony of psychiatrists within the 'mental health' system.

But the other side of the coin is: deinstitutionalization could not possibly have succeeded unless it had established itself on a philosophical basis *other* than the disease model. This would not have been tolerated by the forces committed to maintaining the *status quo.* Deinstitutionalization was a move in the right direction, but it was a toddler's step and when it fell on its face, the most reactionary elements within the psychiatric profession were on hand to recapture control of the American Psychiatric Association and to provide an ideological rationale for the failure of deinstitutionalization.

It failed, they claimed, because it aimed too high. *Madness in the Streets* falsely states that psychotherapy is ineffective with "the chronically mentally ill". Psychiatry's most effective treatments are stated to be psychosurgery, electroshock, and psychiatric "medication". The authors neglect to mention that all these "treatments" are injurious to the brain. (See Peter Breggin's book *Toxic Psychiatry,* 1992.) A massive campaign has already begun to persuade society that individuals who experience distress are genetically defective and incompetent to make decisions about their own treatment. Under the rallying cry of 'the right to treatment' of the 'mentally ill', individuals' democratic rights, including their constitutionally guaranteed right to liberty and to due process of law, will be abrogated. This right includes the right of individuals who do not constitute a danger to themselves or others to be protected from involuntary incarceration in mental hospitals, as well as the right to refuse psychiatric drugs and electroshock.

Madness in the Streets reflects the program and thinking of the 130,000 member organization, National Alliance for the Mentally Ill (NAMI). This organization, which receives funding from the companies that market brain-disabling psychiatric drugs, is comprised mostly of families of 'the mentally ill'. In response to lobbying and public relations by NAMI and hawks within the mental health system, several states have abrogated laws that were enacted in the 1970s in order to protect individuals from psychiatric tyranny. Children, of course, do not have the right to refuse electroshock if their parents so desire. (The APA manual on ECT use, mentioned above, discusses in detail the treatment of young children and adolescents by electroshock.)

For almost two centuries, psychiatrists have been butchering individuals in mental hospitals. Their tortures, termed 'somatic treatments', serve a dual function. On the one hand they provide psychiatrists with a lucrative source of income. On the other hand, they give psychiatrists the appearance in the public eye of being genuine physicians valiantly battling against the epidemic of mental illness.

Similar functions were served by the 50,000 or so lobotomies that were performed in the 1940s and 1950s. As Eliot Valenstein noted in his book on psychosurgery, *Great and Desperate Cures,* "By using these somatic techniques, psychiatrists felt they were brought closer to the mainstream of medicine from which they often felt isolated." This is how psychiatry maintains its hegemony within the mental health system and conceals the fact that individuals suffer not from mental illness, but from real problems that could be alleviated by counselling or by economic and social reforms.

The Myth Of Genetic Defects

Psychiatric propaganda, like *Madness in the Streets,* either states or implies that many individuals have genetic defects that will cause them to develop chronic mental illnesses. But numerous research projects designed to prove that 'schizophrenics' and 'manic-depressives' were doomed by their genes, have failed to do so. David Cohen and Henri Cohen summarized the results of the research: "The only unquestionable result of the twin genetic studies is that they demonstrate the extensive contribution of environmental factors to the etiology of the disorder."

Of course, even this formulation overstates what the genetic studies have demonstrated. All that has been shown is that a particular genotype is correlated with a particular sequence of behaviors. That is, some individuals are predisposed, presumably when under environmental stress, towards manifesting behaviors that are *interpreted* by psychiatrists as 'symptoms' of 'mental illness'. There is no reason to assume that environmental factors cease to operate at the point the psychiatric interpretation is made (or that a disease has taken over the organism).

The strongest of these environmental factors and the most invisible are the baneful interventions of the mental health system that transform an existential crisis into a pretext for what Sarbin and Mancuso aptly termed "the degradation of the individual's social identity."

Instead of facilitating individuals' integration into society, psychiatry, during the period of deinstitutionalization now inducted them into full-time careers as mental patients. Professing the omniscience of the expert, they looked into their scientific crystal balls (such as 'psychodiagnostic' testing) and delivered the judgment 'You have a chronic mental illness.' When their expectations became a self-fulfilling prophecy, they blamed the disastrous results on the 'epidemic of mental illness'. However, the source of the problem lies in the medical model itself which creates and sustains a set of expectations that are fixed, uniform, and low. In this connection, the research on experimental bias is unequivocal. After reviewing the literature on this topic, Jerome Frank wrote in *Persuasion and Healing* (1984), "To recapitulate the chief findings, an experimenter's expectations strongly bias the performance of the subject by means of cues so subtle that neither experimenter nor subject need be aware of them." Furthermore, "A therapist cannot avoid biasing his patient's performance in accordance with his own expectations, based on his evaluation of his patient and his theory of therapy. His influence is enhanced by his role and his status, his attitude of concern and his patient's apprehension about being evaluated." The disease model sustains the expectation that individuals will fail, and consequently it ensures their failure.

In 1980 therapist Jay Haley, who had worked successfully with 'schizophrenics' and their families using a model based on the idea that individuals act crazy in response to unresolved family conflicts, wrote in his classic book, *Leaving Home,* "The main reason I dropped the term 'schizophrenia' was that it so handicapped the teaching of therapy, I found it almost impossible to persuade psychiatric residents—or social workers since they follow the lead of psychiatrists—to expect a schizophrenic to become normal. They would hesitate when they should have pushed for normal behavior and the family would hesitate because the expert did so. Soon everyone was treating the 'patient' like a defective person and therapy failed."

The realities that seem to give substance to the idea of mental illness are created in large part by the mental health system itself. It is the independent environmental variable that transforms acute crises into 'chronic mental illness.' This fact is never even suggested in the mass media. Even leftwing journals, usually critical of genetic rationales for inequality, rarely publish articles critical of the ideology of mental illness.

The complicity of the left in the oppression of 'mental patients' is due in part to the fact that historically progressives in large numbers have chosen to work within the mental health field. It is unfortunate that under the cloak of liberal humanitarianism, many 'progressives' denounce the 'reactionary' Thomas Szasz and demand more money from the government to help the 'mentally ill'.—As if Szasz's defense of laissez-faire capitalism invalidated his critique of psychiatry.

From Madness To 'Mental Illness'

There will be no change unless the idea of 'mental illness' is debunked. We are not dealing with an ontological entity but with an *interpretation* of behavior, an interpretation that serves the interest of the psychiatric establishment, and reassures those who worship at the altar of modern Medicine that we can trust the doctors to save us from the problems engendered by a social order that is disintegrating. Michel Foucault *(Madness and Civilization)* defines the decisive historical moment as "the constitution of madness as mental illness at the end of the eighteenth century." The dialogue between reason and unreason was broken and mad people were rendered mute, robbed of their power to inspire awe and curiosity, demoted in their already marginal social status, and redefined by Medicine as 'mentally ill', to be managed and treated by those with high social status, the medical experts.

The mystery of madness was exorcised. The fascination the mad held for the philosopher, the artist, and the visionary for centuries was written out of the textbooks. This has no place in the annals of psychiatry. It has now been expunged from the popular consciousness by the apostles of the therapeutic State.

How much more profound are the insights of Laing, who argued that "in a society as destructive as our own, going mad may be an adaptive response. It may be that those who do not go mad are less *aware.*" In *The Politics of Experience,* Laing wrote, "The perfectly adjusted bomber pilot may be a greater threat to species survival than the hospitalized schizophrenic deluded that the bomb is inside him." He also wrote, "Only by the most outrageous violation of ourselves have we achieved our capacity to live in relative adjustment to a civilization apparently driven to its own destruction." He dared to develop the thesis, "Madness need not be all breakdown, it may also be breakthrough. It is potentially liberation and renewal as well as enslavement and existential death." This thesis is confirmed by the stories of many of the leaders in the psychiatric survivors movement.

It is corroborated by a transcultural perspective. Julian Silverman in a 1967 article in *American Anthropologist* demonstrated that the initiatory crisis of the future shaman is phenomenologically and behaviorally indistinguishable from the psychotic crisis. However as Silverman notes, "One major difference is emphasized—a difference in the degree of cultural acceptance of a unique resolution of a basic life crisis. In primitive cultures in which such a unique life crisis resolution is tolerated, the abnormal experience (shamanism) is typically beneficial to the individual cognitively and affectively; the shaman is regarded as one with expanded consciousness. In a culture that does not provide referential guides for comprehending this kind of crisis experience, the individual 'schizophrenic' typically undergoes an intensification of this suffering over and above his [sic] initial anxieties". *What were previously interpreted as signs that one was called upon to assume a leadership position in one's culture are now interpreted as symptoms of chronic disorders.*

The Rejection Of The Medical Model

In the past 40 years, on the margins of the mental health system, an exciting new array of approaches to the problems of living have been developed by innovators in the therapy movement. Pioneers in the family therapy movement discovered that by eschewing the medical model and by utilizing a variety of inventive interventions, they were often able to produce dramatic changes in individuals previously considered intractable in brief (six months to a year) periods of time. Cognitive therapists like psychiatrist Aaron Beck provided individuals with the tools to overcome severe depression in three months.

The literature on family therapy is voluminous, although institutional psychiatry has turned a blind eye to it. (Most family therapists, as noted above, have been co-opted by psychiatry.) One characteristic example of a genuine non-medical model approach will have to suffice. Salvador Minuchin was called in as a consultant to a four-person family in which the father had been in and out of mental hospitals for *ten* years and was viewed as severely mentally ill. Minuchin observed the dynamics of the family's interactions and discovered that the man would act incompetent and crazy every time his wife would bring up an issue over which he and she disagreed. Once this dynamic had been identified it took only several months of education, one family session every two weeks, in order to change it. The couple learned to discuss and negotiate conflicts and the man was persuaded of the value of giving up the role he had been encouraged to take on by the mental health experts.

Perhaps the most unusual development (referred to above) was that a number of individuals who had had emotional breakdowns in the late 1960s and 1970s refused to accept the roles of chronic mental patients. Thus, these individuals who had been diagnosed as 'schizophrenics' and 'manic depressives' wrote books; gave lectures; formed self-help groups; organized conferences and demonstrations against psychiatric oppression; and became the pioneers and leaders of the nascent psychiatric survivors movement.

Judi Chamberlin is the most well known of these individuals, partly because her book, *On Our Own,* is an insightful and scathing indictment of institutional psychiatry. Individuals like Chamberlin were empowered by the writings of Szasz and Laing which provided them with an alternative perspective that enabled them to successfully resist the mental health pundits' efforts to help them resolve their identity crises by giving them the identities of 'chronically mentally ill' non-persons.

David Oaks is the editor of *Dendron,* currently the best

antipsychiatry journal in the country. David began school at Harvard in 1973. Over a four-year period David had a number of breakdowns that led to repeated hospitalizations. Yet after each incident, David would resume his education immediately. He ignored mental health experts who told him he was too ill to be in school. He refused to become a chronic mental patient. He graduated *cum laude* in four years. He has not been in a psychiatric hospital or taken psychiatric drugs since his graduation. He is a brilliant social critic, a prolific writer, and a long-time activist both in the psychiatric survivors' movement and the peace and environmental movements.

If the crisis in the mental health system is to be resolved, the disease model must be replaced. The optimal philosophical foundation for any genuine approach to resolving the problems of life is a developmental paradigm or perspective. This perspective engenders positive expectations and consequently does not militate against efforts to encourage education and growth. It is based not on a naive but a mature optimism. It does not deny that people frequently act in ways that are not conducive to their own emotional and spiritual well-being and development; they do this as a result of ignorance, anxiety, confusion, or habit. They may respond to oppression in an unthoughtful or self-defeating manner. It is not that they are ill or defective; they simply do not possess the wisdom, the social resources, the skills, or trust in the environment that would enable them to resolve by themselves the particular life challenges that confront them as individuals. The role of the therapist at its best is not to eradicate an illness but to provide guidance, direction, and emotional support to persons who are involved in a natural process of learning and growth. This process includes existential crises which provide an opportunity for death and rebirth, as Laing noted long ago.

If this change in orientation were effected, which seems impossible now without the mobilization of a mass social movement, the helping profession would be able to help people: it would provide asylum and reassurance to frightened individuals, it would offer individual and family counselling, it would help individuals overcome their addiction to psychiatric drugs that impair their ability to think and create, it would help reintegrate 'mental patients' into society by making available to them education and job training, housing and jobs—it would give them a vision of a future worth struggling for.

Of course, this paradigm shift would mean that therapists would have to address themselves to economic and political obstacles to integrating 'mental patients' into the job market. They would have to become aware of how poverty contributes to emotional distress and interpersonal problems.

They would have to stop presenting therapy as a panacea. As George Albee noted in a recent essay, "Psychotherapy often reveals the human effects of an economic system that produces jobs of incredible boredom and meaninglessness and that periodically throws out of work millions of people who want to work. One out of four preschool children in the

United States is poor and the rate is growing. For them, poverty leads to school failure which in turn leads to crime and delinquency." For their parents it increases the risk of child abuse and neglect. Psychotherapy may reveal this, but Albee continues: "Only when the findings of psychotherapists are translated into well-formulated preventive actions to correct or change the social and economic structure will it have made a significant contribution to prevention."

The disease or medical model impedes individuals' ability to grow and overcome obstacles by attacking at its root their sense of self-respect. It does not recognize the *universality* of the problem, of the human dilemma. The medical model is based on a denial of the fact that every individual is involved in a quest for meaning, happiness and security. It interprets the suffering of individuals who seek psychiatric help as a manifestation of their alleged worthlessness and inferiority.

Even as accomplished and independently minded an individual as Kate Millett was temporarily beaten by the mental health system. In a speech given in 1990 she testified at a gathering of psychiatric survivors: "Remember how you had to truckle before a system which has caused you to suffer and humiliated you nearly to death . . . What do I remember of that time? When I lost my mind to the extent that I believed the nonsense of the medical model, bent my head before unreason, saw myself as the others saw me, as the system saw me, disappeared to myself, expired, vanished as a point of view. I remember this: a sense of the inexplicable in my fate, destiny, sense of doom, helplessness. The fault lay in my genes . . . You knelt down, you capitulated, you said uncle, you swallowed your pride and your self-hood, you bit the bullet and took the pill . . . It was death in life, a half-life, a bondage of the mind in several ways—the mind befuddled with drugs, the mind no longer believed in or trusted. After all, faith in one's own perceptions is one's definition of integrity and wholeness. That was lost. Saddest of all was one's own intellectual honor, its loss."

Kate Millett, it should be noted, finally rejected her official diagnosis of 'manic-depressive' and stopped taking psychiatric drugs more than two years ago.

Psychiatry's New Hardline

In the APA manual *The Practice of Electroconvulsive Therapy* there is scant reference to psychotherapy. No mention is made of any economic or social factors that may cause individuals to become distressed. The pain of heartbreak, the anguish of moral dilemma, the fear of abandonment, homelessness, unemployment, poverty, these do not exist for psychiatry. The cold calculus of pseudo-scientific logic transforms these problems into symptoms of a mental disease that ostensibly will be alleviated by the instruments of medicine. By assuming the guise of medicine, brain injury is legitimized as a major medical treatment.

The APA now seems to be recommending that individuals be subjected to continuous and ongoing electroshock. The manual states that "continuation therapy" (ECT) is "indicated for most patients following completion of the ECT course." The ECT course consists of six to twelve treatments, usually one or two treatments per week. "Continuation ECT should be maintained for at least six months." The document is nebulous regarding the frequency and number of continuation ECT treatment but states: "In many cases treatments are started on a weekly basis with the interval between treatments gradually extended over a month depending upon the patient's response." After continuation therapy is completed, maintenance ECT may be indicated. "In general this frequency will be one treatment per one to three months." Although numerous studies have documented that electroshock causes brain damage, no one has ever assessed the effect on the brain of 20 to 30 years of treatment by ECT.

Critics of ECT have argued that its 'therapeutic' effects were temporary and short-lived. Now institutional psychiatry has conceded the point but instead of seeing this as proof that ECT is at best inadequate and beginning to offer genuine alternatives, it recommends a lifetime course of ECT.

No attempt is made to explain why jolting the brain with electricity and inducing repeated convulsions constitute a treatment for mental illness, which is to say: confusion, loneliness, despair, anxiety. The reason the APA does not attempt to answer this question is because there is no cogent answer that is not incriminating. Critics of ECT have argued that the alleged therapeutic effect of ECT is actually an artifact of the brain damage produced by ECT. In this regard electrically inflicted brain injury is not different in kind from injuries to the brain caused by other forces. In Joseph Wepman's book *Recover from Apasia* (1951), he wrote, "Most brain-injured patients are euphoric. This sense of well-being, lack of concern or anxiety about self, or about anything else, is quite out of keeping with the severity of the patient's problem. He will appear cheerful and largely unconcerned about the condition which the nurse and the doctor recognize as being devastating and debilitating . . . This euphoria may be very disconcerting unless properly evaluated as a typical sign of brain injury. Without euphoria during the early stages of recovery, most patients would be depressed and anxious to the degree that nothing could be done for them. Anxiety and concern begin soon enough, and when it does patients are frequently so upset, so depressed, that only extremely competent handling can induce the motivation to pierce their armor of withdrawal."

John Friedberg, neurologist and author of *Shock Treatment Is Not Good For Your Brain* (1975) stated in a recent interview: "Insults to the brain of any type—strokes, concussions—cause temporary states of euphoria. All neurologists know this. It's no secret. And that's exactly what shock is, a head injury. For a while people feel better, but it's temporary."

Only a mass social movement can counter the increasingly rabid scapegoating of mental patients by the mental health system. The campaign against mental illness deflects attention from the problems that are at the root of the current social crisis. The disease model is an attempt to use the authority of medicine to cloak the realities of inequality and oppression. At a time when racism has lost its legitimacy in many circles as a rationale for inequality, psychiatry is one of the last bastions of those forces opposed to the democratization of the social order. Like the Grand Inquisitor, institutional psychiatry promises security if only individuals will submit to its rule and sacrifice their freedom and dignity. It will suffer its final defeat at the hands of men and women determined to assume the privilege and responsibility of freedom.

Appendix 3
The Network Against
Coercive Psychiatry

Board of Advisors

Stanley Aronowitz, Ph.D., Peter Breggin, M.D., Judi Chamberlin, Phyllis Chesler, Ph.D., Ramsey Clark, George Ebert, Leonard Frank, Kenneth Gergen, Ph.D., Jay Haley, James Hillman Ph.D., Jill Johnston, Ken Kesey, Rev. David Kossey, Cloe Madanes, Jeffrey Masson, Ph.D., James Mancuso, Ph.D., Kate Millett, Ph.D., Kirkpatrick Sale, Dorothy Tennov, Ph.D., Elleen Walkenstein, M.D., John Weakland, Monty Weinstein, Psy.D., Lynn Zimmer, Ph.D.

Board of Directors

Kyle Christensen, Sandra Everett, Seth Farber, Ph.D., Ronald Leifer, M.D., Susan Thornton-Smith.

The Network Against Coercive Psychiatry is an organization comprised of psychotherapists (including psychiatrists), survivors of psychiatric incarceration (commonly known as 'mental patients') scholars and other concerned citizens.

Our position is uncompromising. We believe the 'mental health' establishment has conned the American people.
The idea of "mental illness" is a misleading and degrading metaphor. "Psychiatric treatments" in mental hospitals are for the most part forms of physical and emotional abuse. Psychiatric "diagnoses" are demeaning labels without any scientific validity. The psychiatric Establishment is pushing dangerous drugs which they euphemistically call "medication." Treatments in this century have ranged from revolving chairs to lobotomies to electrical assaults on the human brain to neurologically damaging drugs. There has been no revolution in the treatment of

individuals who are psychiatrically labeled: it is an unbroken history of
barbaric practices, justified by professionals as medical procedures
designed to control patients' ostensible mental diseases.

*The structure of democracy is being undermined by the mental health
system.*
    The Network is emerging at an historical juncture that constitutes a
time of potential danger as well as opportunity. The danger lies in the
continued expansion of psychiatric power and of the merger of the
"mental health" system with the American government. This forebodes
a social control apparatus as totalitarian as that foreseen by George
Orwell in *Nineteen Eighty-Four.* In this case conformity to social norms
would be enforced by mental health professionals playing the role of Big
Brother. The opportunity lies in the possible development of a social
movement against the mental health system.

*For well over thirty years theorists and therapists have been writing
devastating critiques of the medical model of human behavior.*
    Thomas Szasz was the first to argue that to describe individuals who
are having "problems in life" as mentally ill is to use a metaphor that is
misleading and demeaning. It obscures the individuals real problems
and it serves to justify psychiatric coercion and the gratuitous deprivation of individual liberty. R.D. Laing, the British psychiatrist, argued
that 'psychiatric treatment' of 'schizophrenia' typically aborts what is
essentially a natural process tending toward the reconstitution of the self
on a more mature level. Theodore Sarbin and James Mancuso conclude
in their exhaustive study that despite 80 years of popularity, the 'disease
model' has failed to establish its value as either an explanatory theory or
a practical tool. Family therapists like Jay Haley, Salvador Minuchin,
and the Mental Research Institute have demonstrated the extraordinary
success of an approach that is not based on the metaphor of mental
illness. These theorists and practitioners have had virtually no effect on
public policy.

*If the crisis in the mental health system is to be resolved the 'disease
model' must be replaced.*
    Viable models must be based on a developmental perspective.
Psychological and spiritual crises, despair, anxiety, unusual behavior,
and emotional ups and downs are not symptoms of chronic mental
illnesses but natural manifestations of processes of individual and social
growth and maturation. If this change in orientation is effected, the
helping profession will be able to help people: it will provide asylum and
reassurance to frightened individuals, it will offer individual and family
counselling, it will help individuals overcome their addiction to psychiatric drugs that impair their ability to think and create, it will help
re-integrate individuals into society by making available to them

education and job training, housing and jobs—it will give them the vision of a future worth struggling for.

In the absence of this fundamental philosophical change, mental health workers will continue to impede individuals' re-integration into society by branding them 'mentally ill' and by withholding from them opportunities for social and spiritual advancement. The disastrous and unseemly results of the stunting of individual growth by the mental health system will continue to be blamed on 'the tragedy of mental illness'.

A monstrous abuse of power is occurring right now.

The American public is aware through exposure to a variety of documentary materials—including such realistic works of the imagination as *One Flew Over the Cuckoo's Nest* by Ken Kesey—that mental health professionals, in the public sector in another era, abused the authority vested in them. The public has not confronted the fact—and the media have not exposed the fact—that the same kind of monstrous abuse of power is occurring right now. If the radical humanitarian changes advocated by the critics of the mental health system are to be implemented, it will be because the American people begin to realize that they have been abused and mystified by the mental health professions and because they will seize the opportunity to assert their rights and to demand accountability from those who claim to serve them.

People are being tortured, oppressed, and denied ownership of their lives.

Psychiatric survivors have been organizing for human rights and against psychiatric oppression since the mid-1970s. George Ebert, a psychiatric survivor, recently described the reason for his twelve-year involvement in the movement against psychiatric oppression. "As long as the psychiatric state remains, as long as people are being tortured, oppressed, dehumanized, and denied ownership of their lives, we who have survived are obligated to struggle to break the silence." The Network Against Coercive Psychiatry calls upon all socially conscious persons to join the movement.

You can help!

For more information please write or call: Network Against Coercive Psychiatry, 172 West 79th Street, #2E, New York, NY 10024. Or call 212-799-9026.

Index